KIDS IN CRISIS

(Book 1)

–Pediatric ICU 101

Tabitha B. C. Abel

KIDS IN CRISIS –Pediatric ICU 101
Book 1

Copyright © 2019 by Tabitha B. C. Abel

All rights reserved. This book or any portion thereof may not be reproduced or used in any manner whatsoever without the express written permission of the publisher except for the use of brief quotations in a book review.
Printed in the United States of America

First Printing, 2019

ISBN: 978-1689189378

Cover Design by Fiverr.com/ultrakhan22

Weekly Blog Tabel Talk@TabithaBCAbel
www.TabithaAbel.webs.com

DEDICATION

to a wonderful friend and colleague,

gone too soon,

Eleanore Groves.

You are not forgotten.

ENDORSEMENTS

Katherine Dalke, MSN, RN
PICU Nurse Manager (1979-2001)
Loma Linda University Children's Hospital, CA

The KIDS IN CRISIS trilogy is a no-holds-barred peek into the life of a Registered Nurse working in one of the most stressful, challenging, heart-wrenching areas of a hospital – the Pediatric Intensive Care Unit. Abel's incisive writing style reveals the complexity and compassion of the environment with her occasional irreverent humor. Her unique perspective provides the reader with a clear understanding of life in the PICU and how she and her colleagues survived and saved the lives of countless children. Abel's dedication to her work shines through in this book, KIDS IN CRISIS –PICU Nursing 101.

* * *

PJ Koehler, RN
Pediatric ICU Staff Nurse

KIDS IN CRISIS —Pediatric ICU 101 is an interesting, unique book. Tabitha is a gifted writer bringing the world of the PICU Nurse to the forefront, by educating readers who like a true-to-life read. She focuses on true happenings in a PedsICU and shows readers how PICU nurses deal with everyday situations.

The KIDS IN CRISIS trilogy shows how rewarding it is to be that nurse and describes the emotions nurses try to hide in stressful situations, while being strong for the patients and their families. Sometimes they have to go to the Nurse's Lounge for a good cry. I know this to be true, because I am one of those nurses. As a nurse, you give your best —but it doesn't always turn out well for the patient, or their family.

However, when you see a patient that the PICU Team at first gave little hope of a successful recovery, who you took care of for a few months, walking out of the hospital on his own two feet — then tears flow again, but these are tears of joy, because God has worked another miracle in PedsICU.

* * *

Stephen Chavez, Author/Editor
Silver Spring, MD

Tabitha Abel's by-line has appeared often in Adventist Review. I have often had the privilege of editing her manuscripts.

She is a talented writer, and her submissions require little or no editing on my part. This collection of stories is typical of her style: readable, practical, nuanced, and engaging. This book is easy to read and hard to put down. Let her prose transport you as you are introduced to the individuals and situations that have colored her life.

* * *

ACKNOWLEDGEMENTS

KIDS IN CRISIS –Pediatric ICU 101 would not have been published had not many people cheered me on, and believed in me. It has been a long journey. I have worked among amazingly talented, hard-working and diverse colleagues who are focused on our young patients, Our Heroes. Thank you for working with me, helping me through rough times, encouraging me and laughing with me. Also, my thanks to writers, editors and friends who have given me much needed feedback, read chapters for me and encouraged me to keep going.

Some incredible kids and their families made this memoir a reality and many PICU physicians, Respiratory Therapists, Physical Therapists, Chaplains, Social Workers, Child Life Specialists, Unit Secretaries, Transport Team members, and a zillion others who tolerated me, and made PedsICU a brilliant place to work, despite the stress and challenges.

KIDS IN CRISIS –Pediatric ICU 101 is aptly endorsed by: Katy Dalke, a PICU Nurse Manager who directed a large staff with aplomb; PJ Koehler, a colleague of many years and an experienced PICU nurse; and Stephen Chavez, author and editor, who trusted my writing about unfamiliar territory. Thank you so much.

And then there is my family, especially my kids who endured my long work hours and tolerated my wild ideas. Thank you, Todd Cooper, a teacher and musician, and his sweet wife, Yoon; Ross Cooper, our funny guy, and his outgoing wife, Alyssa; and my faithful daughter, Joelle Cooper, a Special Ed teacher who often makes me proud —a chip off the old block some say. Thanks also to my eldest sister, Revel Papaioannou, a retired teacher, who is a sage friend, and to my husband, Gary, for giving me space to finish this project.

Getting KIDS IN CRISIS –Pediatric ICU book in print, has been a miracle –and a marathon, which I could not have accomplished without God's help, who blessed me with a desire –and even talent, to tell these stories.

Thank you.

TABLE OF CONTENTS

DEDICATION

ENDORSEMENTS

ACKNOWLEDGEMENTS

TABLE OF CONTENTS

PREFACE

Ch 1 Happy New Year 1

Ch 2 Report.. 19

Ch 3 Team Players..................................... 39

Ch 4 Chillin'... 65

Ch 5 Surrogates.. 87

Ch 6 Gown Up!... 103

Ch 7 Changing Places 117

Ch 8 Speak Up, I'm Listening 143

Glossary of Terms.. 159

About the Author.. 165

PREFACE

KIDS IN CRISIS is a series of three books about life in a pediatric ICU: children who are critically ill, their families and the medical personnel who provide care to our patients. Each book focuses on different areas of PICU nursing, but overlapping occurs as stories do not fit neatly under each title.

The first book, **KIDS IN CRISIS, Pediatric ICU 101** focuses on the goings-on in a Pediatric Intensive Care Unit (PedsICU, PICU), nurses interacting with and supporting one another, the hierarchy of the team of professionals caring for our kids and some of the challenges a PICU nurse is likely to face at work —with even a little humor. The second book, **KIDS IN CRISIS, PICU Kids, Our Heroes** concentrates on critically ill kids and their stories.

Sad as some of the stories are, each child made a deep impression on me, and our team of caregivers supported the families and one another in many difficult situations. **KIDS IN CRISIS, Families in Crisis,** the third book, focuses on the brilliant families who endure their child's admission to a PICU faithfully, filled with love and compassion –and those who unfortunately do not fall gracefully into this category.

The books are set in Inland Valley Children's Hospital, a fictitious place with a large PICU and pediatric floors. The gathered the stories over a number of years and from various locations. To conceal the identity of the kids, their families and the staff, names have been changed and some are an amalgam of characters. Some details have been changed, although the stories are based on specific occurrences.

Mostly, I wrote the story outlines shortly after they happened and refined and adjusted them over a period of years. The collection grew, and I knew I wanted to pass them on to other nurses and professional colleagues who worked with children in varying capacities, and to parents who had been through the horror of a child's admission to children's hospital. Known to be a little blunt, the stories are bold, and even somewhat raw. Beware. Eventually, after sitting on this manuscript for too many years, it determined to publish the stories as I remembered them. No doubt, not exactly how things happened, but near enough. The backstory of my somewhat weird childhood in England, my life as a parent and student in both the UK and USA, my religious beliefs and faith in God, provide the back-drop for this collection of stories. It is through these lenses that I recall the happening.

.

* * *

As a nurse, we have the opportunity to heal the heart, mind, soul and body of our patients, their families and ourselves. They may forget your name, but they will never forget how you made them feel.

Maya Angelou

* * *

Nursing is not for everyone. It takes a very strong, intelligent, and compassionate person to take on the ills of the world with passion and purpose and work to maintain the health and well-being of the planet. No wonder we're exhausted at the end of the day!

Donna Wilk Cardillo

* * *

CHAPTER 1

Happy New Year

THE ELEVATOR DOORS SLID OPEN and I squeezed in, pushing the number five button without even looking at the array of metal discs to the right of the doors. A purse stuffed with envelopes hung from my shoulder. Each contained the same two sheets of paper – the culmination of plans formulated during sleepless days —and nights, and a driving desire to help decrease the effect of stress and politics felt in my workplace. I hoped my plan would work.

A cover letter told the reader what *Night Light* was about. Most importantly, it would be an organized means of support for our Night Shift nurses when their lives took a downturn and would celebrate their successes, whether in their families, their studies, or at work. We would be prepared, with a little organization. Hopefully, I answered all their questions in the cover letter, and a crisp application form invited them to join *Night Light*. Today, New Year's Day, was a great day to set *Night Light* ablaze.

So often I had looked around the massive medical center and university campus—where I seemed to be a perpetual student, and had been overwhelmed by the fact that each year some student, maybe only one, but at least one —would die suddenly in tragic circumstances. My sister had been that one student more than 20 years earlier, just before Christmas, at another Christian university. Sad thoughts still captured me as each year rolled past. *Who would it be this year? What program would they be in? Or would it be one of our new, young docs?*

HAPPY NEW YEAR

Her sudden death in a pedestrian versus drunk driver auto accident, had been a devastating experience for me. Even now, it was still painful. But then, like many others, I threw myself into my studies and work, to forget the pain. But what about this new year?

I waited impatiently for the eight seconds to pass to get to the fifth floor, and darted through the opening, whipping quickly around the corner. The doors to the pediatric oncology floor were wide open. Glancing up, I saw a bald child on a tricycle with a "Get Well" balloon floating over his head. He was peddling as fast as his legs would go, passing the Nurses Station, and on through the unit. His little legs went like crazy as his bottom hotched from side-to-side on the oversized tricycle.

Cute. The scene epitomized how to be young (and ill) —and yet happy!

The kid's tired mother tried to keep up with him, seeming to enjoy his happiness for a few brief minutes. Perhaps she could forget the endless chemotherapy, radiation, diagnostic tests, nausea, and pain that had been his —and her journey, over the past few months.

I smiled at her, and waved —but she didn't respond.

I'd seen such sights many times before. Cute little kids riding tricycles, or being pulled gently in red wagons among pillows and soft toys. They were usually attached to IV pumps, with large bags of white or yellow TPN swinging back and forth from IV poles, expertly taped to their transportation. At times, vigilant parents stopped to get a familiar staff member to fix their child's annoying pump alarm, even though their child's nurse was the only one who *should* fix it. Some of the kids wore bright knitted hats, while others proudly sported a completely bald pate. *How can I ever think that my life was rough when, no more than yards away from me, families are being torn apart by cancer, or possible death? How selfish can I be?* I thought.

I hurried on, past the pediatric hemoc floor, towards the Pediatric ICU, which was my unit, my second home. For many of our patients and their families, New Year's Day would be a good day. Today they would distance themselves one whole year-number from the desperate trauma of the previous year, hopefully giving them a happy, fresh start to a bright, new year.

But the uncertainty of the future once again struck me. Is life enjoyable for anyone, ever? Is it just an illusion and unattainable? Would this year be different from the last? How many times had I said to myself, *While there is life, there is hope*, only to find that my patient's life had taken a sudden nose-dive? It was a little like my own life. Going along nicely, and then bam... on the verge of disaster. As may happen to others working in critical care, my outlook on life had soured. I had become more pessimistic, hoping for the best —sometimes, but fearing the worst. I knew first-hand what could happen, and it wasn't always good.

I sighed as I walked quickly along the hallway, and through two sets of doors towards the familiar PedsICU, or PICU, as some said. Strangely enough, I loved the excitement of working with the most critically ill kids, and being part of a great team of nurses and physicians (and others), even though, in reality, life in the PICU wasn't as sweet as a bowl of cherries.

The PICU, hidden from prying eyes behind locked doors in the glistening medical center, would become the second home for too many unfortunate families this year. Not because they wanted to discover it, but because they had to. Kids were admitted to the floor, accompanied by parents and grandparents, friends, clergy, social workers, first responders and more. Some adults would enter fearfully, with great trepidation, while others came more boldly, hoping for a miracle. Perhaps their story would have a happy ending —or maybe not. But they could always hope for the best.

"We never thought this would happen to us," Jack's parents had said to me at the end of my last shift –last year. "What would we have done if you, *they meant PedsICU*, hadn't been here? Jack would have never made it if it wasn't for you guys." Jack's parents had come hoping for a miracle, and got it. His recent skateboard accident should have cost him his life —but it hadn't. He would be home this year, in a week or two, wiser, and alive.

Sadly, many others, though, told another story. These families left the PICU with their lives in tatters, for despite the best medical care, their child didn't recover, and PedsICU became the place where they started the long journey from the indescribable pain of losing a child, through the convoluted stages of grief, to an uncertain recovery, and a new phase in their lives.

HAPPY NEW YEAR

They no longer referred to time by the usual nomenclature of day, month and year, but as the day, the week or the month "after Tiffany died" or "after Joseph passed." Life for them was never the same. Life became "after."

It sure was a different world from the Labor and Delivery floor, and even the NICU, or Neonatal Intensive Care Unit. Both departments I knew well. But now, PedsICU was home to me. It was my world. But today, I hadn't come to the PICU to work —even if the staffers pled with me to work a shift. It was unlikely, because it was January 1st, and while some nurses coveted holiday time to be with their family, others fought to work holidays because they got time-and-a-half pay. No, I was on a different mission.

Slowing my pace, I neared the PedsICU because, like on many other days, people huddled in clusters outside the double doors of the unit, and I could not barge into them. It looked ominous, and a heavy feeling came over me. Forget the excitement of a new year. No one would know it was January 1st if they looked at the congested hallway (even at this early hour).

I knew it —but hopefully, I was wrong. *Please, God, I hope I'm wrong.*

* * *

I shoved my badge in the card slot to open the doors, pushing on the double-doors while hoisting my bag onto my shoulder, and slid through the doors. Inside, a small group of people stood with their arms around each other. The younger adults were in their late thirties, and a tall, distinguished man, with thinning grey hair, stood among them.

"I can't believe he isn't going to make it," I heard a tearful woman in the group whisper, as I passed by.

"We must have faith," spoke up another. I was right. It was bad.

An overweight man leaned against the wall, alone, staring out of the picture-windows on the other side of the hallway. He didn't move as I passed him.

Happy New Year, I thought in disgust as I reached the secretary's desk. So much for a Happy New Year. How stupid could I be to think that a Happy New Year was ever possible here? Duh!

HAPPY NEW YEAR

I walked on, and opened the mailroom door.

***

Candy, one of the AM Charge Nurses, sat in front of the computer entering the patient acuities for the shift, a necessary duty to adequately staff the floor for the next shift.

Candy was an energetic, unconventional woman who would take a 20-mile bike ride over rugged terrain for fun. For fun! She took part in bike clinics in her spare time, and had almost completely bounced back after a severe back injury resulting from a fall from her bike on a narrow mountain trail a while ago. Candy had an explosive, spicy, upbeat personality with aptness to burst into spontaneous laughter at the slightest provocation. And, at only 5 feet 2 inches, she could stand up for herself.

Once, a towering Pediatric Resident wrote an incorrect order on the Physician Order Sheet, and she confronted him asking, "And just what do you think you are doing? Are you crazy?" Taken aback by her questions, as many had been before, he checked his orders and wisely corrected them. The Attending then took the Resident aside, and told him that he'd better listen to the nurses —especially Candy, if he wanted to make it through his Residency. Sage advice. He learned well, and passed the information on to his colleagues.

The other Charge Nurses had strong personalities too, and were not to be "messed with" either. But Candy's slightness, and the panache with which she delivered her rebuffs (or advice), made her comments extra poignant. More than once she'd been heard saying, "Today this is my unit, TODAY, and I'm not called Charge Nurse for nothing! Do you get it?" Then she'd laugh.

The kids came first, but when Candy's nurses were being spoken down to by one of the physicians, they had better watch out. Her nurses would be shown respect by the physicians on her watch —and by the patients' families too. She might be only five foot two, but she was a raging fireball when ignited.

Candy's downside though, was her handwriting. It was an utter disaster and caused some good-natured comments. But Candy didn't care. She would laugh it off saying, with a huge grin, "Take a lesson in reading," and that was the end of the matter. At least Candy never complained about physicians' handwriting! It was fortunate that she entered the acuities into a computer, and did not write the numbers down on paper, for who could tell how many staff would be scheduled for the next shift had she written them by hand! Engrossed in what she was doing, Candy didn't look up as I started to read the names along the staff's mailboxes.

"So, what's happened to that family Candy?" I asked, as I continued checking the names. There were more than 80-mailboxes, and most of the night staff's boxes were on the upper level. I knew Candy could not give me all the facts, due to HIPAA, but I got her attention, and she looked up.

"It makes me mad. It's the usual crap," Candy said, not waiting for me to comment. "When will they ever learn? Hospitals screw up. What's new? Hell, am I mad!"

Candy didn't often swear, but she did not take screw-ups lightly either.

"Here we are again; trying to pick up the pieces after the damage is done. Not before, mind you, *after*. Diabetes again."

"A new onset?" I asked.

"Nope," Candy replied succinctly, never one to waste words. "'Been one for five years. It should have never happened." She paused adding, "But this is his first admission since diagnosis. Sometimes I want to wring those doctor's necks!" Her eyes flashed. She was ready to fight anyone who disagreed with her, and I knew better than to do that. "Why don't they learn how to treat kids? Don't they realize kids aren't adults?" She caught her breath. "Let me get my hands on them!" She was on a roll, so I said nothing.

"The kid was ill, and the docs misdiagnosed him. They checked him out in their ER and sent him home. The kid didn't get better, and the parents thought that *they* were the stupid ones." She paused, and her voice softened. "So, the parents wasted more time thinking they must be mistaken. You can't blame the parents. They did what they thought was right. But sometime later, they took him back to the ER still with a sky-high blood glucose. It was much worse than before." Her voice trailed off.

"Don't those docs know how to treat kids? Of course not," she answered herself sarcastically. "They panicked, and dropped his blood sugar w-a-y down, and called Doc Mike and the Transport Team." She paused. "What a mess. It makes me sick!"

I guessed the worst. "He herniated? ... Is he gone?"

"Yeah, well ... as good as."

Candy's energy had fizzled out. She leaned back on the chair. "What gets me is that this is the second botched-up job in the last six months. We need to get the message out somehow. I know they are doing their best—but it isn't good enough."

I nodded. "The team flew, didn't they?" I asked.

"Yeah, but we were too late. The kid herniated soon after the they got there," she said. "It's just a matter of time—and today of all days," Candy groaned.

"If only we could catch things before it's too late. We need our docs to get out to the boonies –and educate those ER docs." Calming down, Candy added, "The truth is that this kid was probably the first child that ER doc had seen in his life with a blood sugar like that."

"Candy," I interjected, "I heard the family talking about faith as I passed by. Do you think they would donate? I mean, something good could come out of this mess. It is the New Year after all." She was quiet. "It would be a great way for other families to start their year," I added.

"Yep, Tabitha. We're already on to that." She paused. "We're hopeful."

The local Organ Procurement Agency for Southern California was notified as soon as a child started to plummet to a level that survival might be in question. Their staff was a team of professionals who were not employed by the medical center, and who could answer every question a family would ask about organ donation. They approached the families and gave them ample time to make the right decision for their family to live with, for the rest of their lives. The Agency did an excellent job in procuring, and placing much-needed organs around the south-western States.

I reached into my bag and placed an envelope containing an application form in Jacqui's and Daniel's mailboxes —and then into every night nurses' mailbox. *Night Light* would require a small monthly membership fee which would provide cards and small gifts for staff as they experienced their personal emergencies. My theory was that if there were funds on hand, and cards and simple gifts, *Night Light* would always be ready to support our colleagues when their lives hit "a bump in the road". We could take action right away, and make them feel that we, the *Night Light* team (their colleagues), really cared about them. That might help them get through their difficult time. Those of us who were ready to pull a joke on someone else (in good fun), or were willing to laugh at ourselves, could develop the fun side of *Night Light*. Hopefully it would decrease everyone's stress levels, and boost our endorphins at the same time. It was worth a try. I shot the last envelope into Nila Yadzinski's box and, with my mission accomplished, turned to Candy. "It's too bad Candy. Today of all days."

I made my way out of the unit, turned right and walked past the family once again. The lone man gazing out of the window, was still staring outside, as if mesmerized by the waving palm fronds fluttering in the bright, blue, winter skies. Matchbox-sized cars rushed helter-skelter along the freeway, west towards Los Angeles, and east towards Palm Springs and the Arizona border. A network of bridges to the west carried traffic from the High Desert south towards the smoggy basin of the inland cities, and on towards San Diego and the Mexican border. Every route moved busy people going somewhere —fast; oblivious as to what had happened today to his grandson.

He stood stock-still. Waiting for time to pass—but that too had stopped, right on New Year's Day.

A lady wept quietly, comforted by emotionally stronger people, or perhaps people less closely related to the child. They were all in a state of shock, even as the pain began to sink in. It would be a long, long time before their lives would be joyful again. Sadly, complete healing would never happen. They had lost an irreplaceable child, and life had changed forever. Three hundred and sixty-five days had to pass before they could move themselves from the year when everything changed.

My heart ached for them. Beneath my down-to-earth, brusque exterior, I had a heart that responded to the pain of others. We knew our work was often downright heart-wrenching, but my trust and dependence on God gave me the strength to cope with the challenges. The loss of this life though, on New Year's Day, reminded me of the delicate cross-stitch, wall-hanging displayed in the hospital hallway, which no doubt had been made by a grateful parent. It read, "Life is Precious, Handle it with Prayer."

How true.

The elevator doors opened, and I stepped inside, escaping from the grieving family. At lobby level I hung a left, and headed for the crisp winter air. Blinking in the bright light, I breathed in deeply and counted my blessings—three healthy kids, and a moderately comfortable life. This year I would have hundreds of yet-unknown opportunities to make a difference in the lives of many kids, and their families—and in my colleagues' lives too. One of my New Year's resolutions was already underway. All the night staff had been invited to join *Night Light*. Now I had to wait and see if it would have the desired, positive effect. Today could, after all, be the start of a good year for me.

CHAPTER 2

Report

THE AFTERNOON SUN WINKED through heavy, dark green curtains putting my mind slowly into gear. I was tired. My body still ached as I turned and buried my face in the pillow. I would grab another 15-minutes. But I didn't –or did I?

My eyes shot open with the loud drilling of my alarm clock. It was 3 PM, and I had 25-minutes to get to school to pick up my daughter. I opened the "morning" devotional at my bedside, dropping it open to today's reading. "I look to you, heaven-dwelling God, look up to you for help, Psalm 123:1". How right. I knew I couldn't keep myself and the family on track unless I had a Higher Power to call upon, and for me that was God. He was my Helper. However, with that godly thought in my mind, I did what I so often did. I asked for His guidance throughout the next day —or rather night, and for God to protect my children and a cousin who was battling cancer, and then threw in an offer of commitment to Him (as if He needed me to do that), and was in the shower before I could finish my prayer with an Amen.

In one way it was reassuring to know that God knew my innermost thoughts and intentions, but it also made me feel uncomfortable as my busy schedule forced me to limit my time with God. That was another lie. I made my own choices and needed to get my act together, and stop making excuses. These thoughts tweaked my conscience, but I buried them in the back of my mind. I would revisit them another time—probably tomorrow, when I did the same thing again. However, one day, I would make some lasting changes, perhaps.

REPORT

By the time three hours had passed, I had done the impossible. First, I had picked up my daughter from school (on time) and then baked chocolate chip cookies from scratch. I made spaghetti and salad for the family for dinner, packed my sack lunch, fed the dog, tangled with 8th-grade mathematics and signed the parental consent form for my daughter's field trip to the Civil War Costume Museum tomorrow. I gave her $10 to spend in the gift shop and left instructions with my husband as to what time she had to be at school in the morning —and then got ready for work.

Three cookies were missing from the cookie-sheets by the time I scooped up the humongous, soft-baked cookie that lay on a baking-tray alongside a calligraphed sign saying "Do not touch." Signs must look beautiful, I thought, and being rushed should not ruin my calligraphy. It was also the only way I could be sure I would get the message over to my three, "starving" children. This particular cookie was laden with chocolate chips that were begging to be devoured, and would have disappeared without a trace had I not made a prominent sign.

"And where is that going?" my husband asked as I carefully lifted the cookie onto the middle of a paper plate.

"To work," I replied. "I think Leah could do with that cookie more than you guys."

They all knew that. If and when I baked cookies, the biggest and best cookie went with me to work, leaving them to drool at the thought of missing the best culinary specimen of the batch! "Might have known that," he mumbled.

I left 20-minutes early for work. Like the night before, I was in charge —something that I did as one of a small band of Relief Charge Nurses. When neither of the two regular Night Charge nurses was scheduled, one of the group was scheduled. That meant I had to be at work in enough time to find out how the patient-load looked, and divvy-up the lists.

* * *

Dropping my backpack on the floor in the Report Room, I carefully slid the cookie into Leah's mailbox. There would be a few changes on the floor tonight, as was almost always the case. Hopefully all the scheduled

REPORT

staff would turn up, and it would be a fantastic night. Some hopes. More likely, it would be a matter of surviving a 12-hour shift of routine, exasperating nursing care, with a heavy sprinkling of challenging situations for us, and a living nightmare for up to 25-families.

The Report Room was empty, but the unit secretary, whose shift started 10-minutes earlier, had organized her space nearby and was ready to rock-and-roll her way through the next 12-hours.

"Can you call Candy for me Connie? She must be somewhere out on the floor," I called to her.

Sitting down, I started to digest the Shift Report while I waited.

It was much like the night before except for a few changes. There were three empty beds right now, and an 18-month-old trauma case was in Room 1 where Joanna, the 30-day-old kid with meningitis had been the night before. She had been transferred to the Step-down ICU. *Wonderful news.*

I looked more carefully along the new kid's report: intubated, neuro checks stable, head CT negative, *excellent*, but fractured orbits and sinuses, *ouch…that couldn't feel good.* I turned a page, and my eyes lit on a penciled-in name. Vanessa Abbott —spider-bite being transported from the desert. *Hmmm...that must be one big bad spider.*

* * *

Candy was on the floor, somewhere, embroiled in trying to persuade Terri to stay over until 3 AM. Terri was one of a few nurses who were reasonably flexible with her time, and she was often willing to stay over, or come in early.

"I'm not asking you to come in early tomorrow Terri," Candy cajoled. "No, I need a kind nurse," she said pretending to be suddenly hit by a new thought, "like you for instance," she said with a brightening smile. As if the message hadn't gotten through, she added, "to stay over a few hours until Kathleen comes in at 1 AM. You would be home by 2 AM –if not before. I would really appreciate your doing that for me, and of course, Tabitha would love you for it, too."

Candy paused. Timing was everything.

"I would be very grateful," she repeated, snapping on her sweetest smile.

REPORT

Terri was stoic. Candy's sweet-talking voice dripped with honey, but it didn't work. Terri had plans. She was going shopping tomorrow with Arlene, and no amount of begging would make her change her plans. No way.

Candy saw she wasn't making headway, so she tried another angle.

"Well, I think I could squeeze a couple of hours out of Kathleen and get her in at eleven tonight to relieve you. Would that work for you?" she persisted, weighing each word carefully.

Terri wavered.

"Pretty pleeeease?" Candy wheedled. "I'll make it up to you next time you and I are on… I'll give you the pick of the one-to-one lists…I promise."

Terri had to decide. Four hours at time-and-a-half would mean extra dollars and, if she went home on time, she probably wouldn't go to bed before eleven o'clock anyway. Also…the night staff was in a bind, and she tried to help out where she could. Terri was a sucker for that, and everyone knew that. What to do? Keep working? "Okay."

As soon as "okay" was out of Terri's mouth, Candy slapped her jovially on the back, thanked her, gave her a huge grin and headed for the Charge Nurse's office.

"I owe you," she said as she turned to leave. "I knew I could rely on you."

I was still scanning the 5-page document when Candy opened the door, taking it almost off the hinges. She headed straight for her swivel chair and slumped down into it.

"Connie, call Kathleen and see if she will make it for eleven. If she won't, we're screwed!" Cindy barked. She turned to me. "Phew! I don't know about me owing Terri a favor, but you owe me one now. I thought she would never agree to stay over!"

"Maybe you are losing your charm Candy," I replied, "or perhaps everyone has learned to read you like a book! But thanks, I'm sure it'll work out. It's not your problem now."

"No, and I did my best." She flashed a smile. Known for finagling favors, Candy was not ashamed of today's compromised success with Terri.

REPORT

"Do you think Kathleen will come in at eleven for a 20-hour shift?" I asked, fearing the worst, but hoping for the best.

"No," she said springing up in her chair. "She had agreed to one o'clock when I last spoke to her."

"What about Craig or Kirsten? Is either of them on? They're always worth a try," I asked.

"'Fraid not. I guess you will have to leave it in the capable hands of staffing!" she joked. "Or you could pray. It's a whole lot better than relying on the staffers to make the calls!"

"Perhaps the Supe will give us a Resource Team nurse for a couple of hours, or we'll get Connie to call the day nurses before they go to bed —at least the ones who are likely to agree to come in early. Whatever…"

Connie interrupted Candy and me by yelling from her desk, which was less than 10-feet away, at the front of the unit. "I heard you, Tabitha. I just got tomorrow's schedule. I'm on it. Slave drivers! I barely get here, and you're cracking the whip!"

Candy rolled her eyes and, unconcerned by Connie's comments, turned her attention to her old, scribbled-on Report Sheet. She was ready to give me the down-and-dirty before we assigned the lists to the night nurses. Candy wanted me to hand out the lists pronto.

"What's up with this spider-bite, Candy? Do you know when the kid will be here?" I asked. "Is she going into Room 10 or 19? Her name's written in both places?"

"Nineteen," Candy promptly replied. "Sorry, it got a bit crazy–as usual."

Candy slumped down further into her seat, and stuck her legs out in front of her with a much-used copy of the Report Sheet held aloft. "By the way, I sure am glad to see you!" she said looking up at me. "I am so ready to go home!" Candy was always ready to go home, so that was no surprise, but maybe today had been worse than usual.

"I've had crap from parents –and doctors, up to here," she exploded, slicing her hand across her forehead. "Then, if that's not enough, Myrna called in sick–late, of course, right after the transport call. And by the way, that spider-bite won't be here for another hour.

REPORT

They called back about 15-minutes ago and said she was "fine"–only some abdominal pain and climbing up the wall —so they've given her some Ativan® to calm her down. Sweet! But everything is okay, and I've even set up nineteen for you. Left it as an odd."

I rechecked the Report Sheet. Station Four already had three one-to-ones and now the "fine" spider-bite as well? If another kid came in later, it might go well with the spider-bite, but if the next admit was really bad, what would I do? There was little room for maneuvering patients around the floor–and getting two admissions wouldn't make a nurse happy. But then perhaps no patient would be admitted after the spider-bite, and whoever got it would have a great night. It might even be the best list! Who could know? No one had a crystal ball.

"You're using 14-nurses —and Terri is keeping her list for the time being. You have one NICU nurse floating here. I have written her name by Rooms 2 and 4. I think they'll be the best for her. Little kids–respiratory distress in Room 2 with a trach, and Ivan in four, with apnea and pneumonia. He's less than a month–so she should be happy."

Carefully I re-counted the names written on the staffing list. Then, picking up the assignment cards, the staffing list, the report sheets, and a pen, I proceeded to open the door anticipating I may —or may not, be eaten alive by the night staff. The unit was already bulging at the seams with critically ill kids, and it looked as though it could be a crazy shift.

"Let's hope everyone is here," I said to Connie as I passed by her desk. "I sure don't want any extra hassle tonight."

Connie gave me a knowing smile and, not missing a beat retorted, "Neither do I. But you don't seem to realize that yet!"

I head-counted the nurses in the Nurses Lounge and sat down. None of the scheduled nurses were missing. *What a relief.* "Thanks, everyone for being here," I said. "I am hoping for a great night tonight. Got a spider-bite coming in soon, and so far, nothing's in the pipeline." Smiles all around.

The NICU nurse took her list without complaint, and three nurses were back from the previous night. Two of them kept their assignments, and the other nurse

REPORT

took the new head-injury, trauma kid in Room 1. The remaining nurses then went into a "smash and grab" mode, checking names with diagnoses, and other details, and once they had made their choice, writing their names on the Report Sheet next to their patient's names. All but one list was taken.

"Who hasn't got a list?" I called out. Premila, a quiet, efficient, no-trouble nurse, waved her hand in the air. In no hurry to pick a list, she had decided to avoid the scrum and see what she got.

"Well Prem, I guess you're the lucky nurse to get Michelin Man in Room 5. He's an odd —but there's nowhere to admit, so you should be okay. You know Keith anyhow, don't you? The huge kid with Prader-Willi?"

Prem nodded.

"You'll do a great job," I cooed. "And Prem … if you need help, call me. You don't have to struggle with him on your own."

The nurses started to pick up their stuff, and the chatter began. "Hold it guys," I bellowed. "Anyone for prayer? No devotional tonight...sorry, but we sure could use a prayer. It's going to be busy."

Nurses who did not go to church routinely respected those who believed in God and prayer. There was quiet, but no one volunteered to pray. "Okay guys, I guess it's me. Let's pray. "Dear God, we ask for your presence with each one of us tonight, and with our kids and their families. Help us to do our best –and bless our families at home. We are Your hands, and in Your hands. Amen." We didn't have to pray, but most Charge Nurses did before we set out. It made an excellent start to the shift, and was unifying.

"Amen" rippled through the room as everyone picked up their bags and started to file out of the Nurses Lounge chatting quietly in anticipation of another long, busy shift.

I gathered up the papers in one hand, thankful that there had been enough nurses for the patient load. It had gone smoothly so far, and I had a great team of nurses to work with again. *Thank you, Lord.*

I ambled back into the Report Room to get a full report from Candy. I knew that she would go through

REPORT

the report like a freight train, so, with pen poised and the report sheets listing location, name, diagnosis, and physician in front of me, I got ready for the rush.

"Okay," Candy started barely looking up to see if I was ready or not. "Here's the deal. Station One. Looks as though it will be okay. Room 1's the new trauma – intubated, somehow got hit in the face when his brothers were playing baseball in the park. Looks a real mess –but he'll be okay. Surgery went well. He'll need quite a bit of sedation. Parents are cool. If all goes well, he'll be extubated in the morning. No problems with the respiratory distress kid in Room 2. He's keeping his feeds down. Room 3's another new kid. Came from out west somewhere, with a left pleural effusion. He got here about three, and all the admitting stuff is done. Really nice parents, but they're freaked out." She paused momentarily. "Should do okay. He's a one-to-one at the moment, but if you have to, you could put him with Keith in (Room) 5, and Prem could take an admit somewhere else."

She hurried on. "On Station Two there's a 7-year-old with ALL who's not doing too well —really busy, a one-to-one. In Room 7, there's that 16-month-old with pneumonia on the vent. A bit of a puzzle. I never got to read his history, but they did a sweat chloride test for Cystic Fibrosis. Room 9's a 12-year-old having reconstructive facial surgery in the morning. Usual pre-op stuff. He is going to OR early tomorrow. Next is an empty bed."

Candy was on a roll. She'd had a long day, and nothing was going to stop her from going home ASAP, if not before.

"Station Three is a mess," she said. "Cute little Anna is still on the vent. You remember her, don't you?" Candy didn't wait for a reply. "She's the 2-month-old with Dandy-Walker." I nodded my head. I really did remember Anna. She was the cutest little thing ever.

"Next is Pedro. You remember him? Three months old. He was very busy all day and will be tonight. He's still on the vent, and needs a blood transfusion before going to surgery in the morning. His chances aren't good in the long run, but he'll do okay this time around. Next to him is the ruptured appy. ALOC on tons of antibiotics. I've paired him with Adam in (Room)14, next door. No change in him. His shunt was revised today – again. He's doing well so far." She flipped the page over

REPORT

to Station Four —and then turned the page back again, clearing her throat loudly. The train had screeched to a halt.

"Not forgetting, of course, the last kid on Station Three," she laughed, "a 21-monther who is severely dehydrated." And then, picking up speed again Candy continued. "That's enough about him. Only two stations to go."

"Station Four," she said as if reading a shopping list. "Room 16 is a newly diagnosed AML. Fifteen-years-old. He's pretty busy–but doing okay. It's a bad age to be hit with leukemia…well, any age is bad, but at 15 you're not really a kid, and yet you're scared spitless by it all. Sad."

She paused as I nodded in agreement. It *was* a bad age to have leukemia.

"Room 17 is Mackey. MVA kid, intubated, but going to do okay. Then there's a 4-monther, Mendoza, with seizure disorders due to metabolic problems. He's also on the vent," she added.

"Station Five is no better, sorry. A 13-year-old playing asinine games ended up as a closed head trauma with a fractured pelvis. What silly buggers kids can be!

They think they're untouchable at that age. He's still in spinal precautions, and hates being log-rolled."

Not wanting to lose momentum, the freight train raced towards the final stop.

"Room 23's has the 8-year-old with a fractured femur in traction. He's doing okay. Nothing new with him, but we've got a new one in 24. He's 5-years-old, Marcus. He was riding pillion on a motorbike when it hit a wall!" she laughed. *Good grief.* "The kid was wearing a helmet, thank God. His brainless dad was up front and got a few cuts and bruises. He's feeling pretty guilty though."

"So he should. I would like to pinch his head off!" I interjected.

Ignoring me, Candy continued. "Marcus has frontal fractures, jaw fractures and his right foot is fractured. And finally," she said catching her breath, "–there's Mandy with the astrocytoma. Eight years old. She's had a bad day today. She is one sad little case. I don't know how her parents are dealing with this. Finished," she shouted triumphantly standing up and slamming the Day

REPORT

Report Book shut on the table, crushing the Report Sheets between its pages.

"THE END. I'm off duty. Don't call me if you need me!" Candy said with a laugh, and left. *Of course she would be back the next day! We all came back for more.*

I sat back in my chair. Too many sad little people and their families. There was a lot of pain, but also hope, and being hopeful, and positive, and upbeat was still my resolution, even if it was no longer the New Year. I pondered what the most pressing need was for now.

"I'm going to check on the Float," I said to Connie. "Have you found anyone to relieve Terri?"

"Patience, Tabitha," Connie scolded. "I'm still trying."

Tonight was no different from any other shift. Kids in pain, parents devastated by their kid's illness, nurses doing their best to care for their patients. No wonder PICU nurses are stressed. Stressed almost every day, but bored —never.

PEDIATRIC ICU 101

CHAPTER 3

Team Players

A WIDE VARIETY OF PATIENTS is admitted to the PedsICU both in age (between a day old and 18-years) and diagnosis. In time, nurses develop a preference for certain types of patient. The system the night staff used in our PICU to get their list of patients for the next shift, allowed us to seek patients we felt were a good match for ourselves. Nurses returning after their first shift usually kept the patients they had the night before, if the patients were still there, or, they might want to avoid a certain child and get a "better" list when they returned for their second night.

When I was very young, my parents divorced. It made little difference to me as my father lived in India, and I lived in England. However, he had the camera and when he left, the camera went too. Our last family photographs were taken when I was almost a year old. My parents, and all five of us children were together. Later, when I was almost five years old, someone took two photos of my sister Rebecca, and me. England is not known for its long summers, but on the one day of summer that year, we lined up our soft toys on chairs and blankets, outside, on the lawn. We posed with them and voila – a visual memory in the photo album. Perhaps that was my first expression of organizing something. My toys were appropriately set out by size and type! Maybe I had inherited the organization skill from my father, who was a Bank Manager for the Bank of India. He must have had a penchant to be organized. I don't recollect my mother making anything other than a weekly shopping list.

By the time my daughter had grown up, she took it as a compliment when an aunt told her that she was like her mother, because she was "so organized" in getting everything planned and done. So, I will grab that as a compliment too.

I had my system to select patients for my shift, especially if it was my first night to work. Other nurses prioritized their choices in their selected manner, whatever that might be. I was not particularly interested in selecting a list for the shift according to diagnoses, which I mentally organized by systems, such as being diseases of the respiratory, cardiovascular or neurological system, or from categories such as trauma, NAT, congenital disorders etc., but rather, I first cast my eyes over the age categories: infants, toddlers, elementary school-age children or, the dreaded, teens. My favorite category? Teens, or as near to that as I could get. Mouthy. Rebellious. Angry. Or, just maybe, really nice, well behaved adolescents. It didn't matter. They were my first choice and the busier the list, the better. Being busy made the shift fly by quickly, and kept me engaged.

* * *

I worked the night shift because I had a busy life – school, children and home, and it somehow enabled me to squeeze a few more hours into a 24-hour day.

Most nurses love to spend money -and need to pay bills, and therefore must earn it as quickly as possible. They like the fact that full-time work is three 12-hour shifts a week. Nowadays, there is little downtime at work, as the health-dollar is being squeezed to get every last drop of blood out of every cent, and budget cuts and declining health-dollars make bedside nursing often extremely stressful and exhausting. But there is pay-back for working full-time in the clinical setting of a hospital. It is four, glorious days (or nights) off work, each week. These can sometimes be attached to the next week's shifts off duty, and hey-presto, a mini-vacation without using vacation time.

The nursing dress code is also inviting. How many workers who meet the public in their workplace, do so wearing pajamas? But nurses might as well call their scrubs, pajamas. They are comfortable, and cute –and, if necessary, can be night attire. Now many hospitals require a certain color of scrubs for different staff types, with good reason, but in the past it wasn't so.

Like many nurses, I was also in school —postgraduate school, and that was challenging. Too often, I found myself propping my eyes open at an 8 AM class after a hectic 12-hour shift, and hearing lectures wax and wane as I slowly succumbed to sleep —for a minute, or two, or even three. At times, I was so desperate for sleep after leaving work, that I drove to the campus, slept in my car for twenty or thirty minutes, only to be awakened by my phone alarm. Then, I had to wake up and focus immediately, so that I could cross the parking lot safely and stumble into the right classroom. It was challenging. However, somehow I managed to get there on time, and alert enough to give the illusion that I could concentrate and participate in the discussions. Sadly, being spry did not last for a full hour, and the need for sleep became overwhelming as I drifted into the head-bobbing zone of fuzziness where nothing made sense. But many nurses did this, and I was a glutton for punishment. I went to bed late when I wasn't working, and rose early to run, go to class or study, or to just get on with packing as much as I could in the day. Later, when I had enough degrees securely stashed under my arm, I took an adjunct faculty position at a nearby college, and the nurse-staffers willingly worked with me to accommodate my complex schedule.

It was life, my life, and I loved it –most of the time. My kids were healthy and busy with school, music, church, and sports, and, as time passed, they left home for further education –or not, as the case maybe, and despite the challenges, God blessed me. I tried never to overlook His abundant blessings and watch-care.

I loved adventure, and a shift on PedsICU could be that! Being paid for it was a plus, and I worked with a team of great nurses, physicians and other healthcare providers. Working allowed me to pay my mortgage, keep food on the table and clothes on my kids' back, and to keep them in Christian schools. Luxuries also became a possibility. Occasionally a group of the PICU staff went to Las Vegas by bus, but my down-time included training for, and then entering road races which were getting costlier every year. Hiking the trails in the magnificent Pacific Northwest was cheaper, but took more planning and time, and included the inevitable expense of travel, motels or campsites. Of course, I dreamed about trips home, to England –but those rarely happened. However –I was a sucker for extra shifts. *Yes, siree, sign me up for another shift. I'm ready.*

TEAM PLAYERS'

* * *

It was mid-May and almost 7 PM, time for the night shift to begin. I wriggled into my wild-animal, nurse's uniform-top, pulled on a pair of plain, dark-blue pants and added yellow, fluorescent socks to the mix. They matched the yellow tigers on my top. My off-white shoes looked as though they should become gardening shoes before the month was out, but I was ready for another night. Anything could happen in the next 12-hours, and that's what kept me coming back.

The nurses piled into the Nurses Lounge. It was a large room with a television in one corner which was bolted to a sturdy platform, and stood almost seven feet off the floor. The TV was rarely off, providing a never-ending, background-noise. I wasn't in charge and I hoped the shift would be ordinary.

Nurses sat around a large table beside bulging bags filled with essential items for the shift. There were lunch bags and snacks, bottles of water containing bobbing ice blocks, big-gulp mugs with lids —to comply with OSHA regulations, clipboards and stethoscopes, study books or magazines -just in case, calculators to confirm medication dosages according to each child's weight, personalized shift report sheets, and more. The days of everyone having a smartphone were in the future, so many nurses chatted as they waited for the shift to begin. The noise increased as more nurses arrived, and spoke louder, to be heard above the din.

Leftover lunch items and napkins from the previous shift littered the center of the table. Taped to the wall over the sink, read a sign, "Clean up your mess, you pigs! I'm not your mother!" Who could have written that? A small group of nurses chatted around a smaller table, while others sat on soft padded chairs chaotically lining the lounge's perimeter, probably left in disarray by the previous shift. Nurses were here to work, not to clear, or clean, the room. And so, the disorder remained untouched as the television droned on, unwatched.

I barged through the door. "What's up?" I enquired to no one in particular as I dropped my heavy backpack on the table and pulled a seat up behind me.

Suzette was the first to answer. With a mischievous smile she replied, "Well, I'm here. We had two admits a while ago," she cooed, "and two bad traumas are coming," she added, in case we had overlooked her news. "That means," she paused, "I don't have to float tonight. It's my lucky night!"

"You should be ashamed of yourself Suzette," I joked. Nurses nearby smiled and laughed at my comment.

"It may be your lucky night, but I'm sure it's not theirs," someone quipped.

At slack times, the excitement of a bad trauma, or near-death situations gave PICU nurses a lift. The adrenaline rush brought with it amnesia as to the reality of the catastrophe that the patient and his family were experiencing.

"Well, Suzette didn't cause the accident," a nurse retorted, "did she?" She paused. "And we'd be out of a job if there were no MVAs!" She was right and, in a twisted way, PICU nurses were the beneficiaries of someone else's nightmare.

It was good that Suzette was working tonight. She was a great nurse with a lot of experience, whose life was never dull. Suzette lived an active, out-door life, often hiking, back-packing or getting caught in unusual situations with her family. She was now a Per Diem

Nurse, and was therefore paid at a higher rate than the regular crew. The downside of being Per Diem was that she would be the first to float to another unit if the census was low, or if the floor was fully staffed with regular PICU nurses. Having to float frequently to another unit was off-putting to many nurses. They would naturally like the higher rate of pay and flexible schedule of being Per Diem, but floating often was too high a price to pay. But, when Suzette walked in the door for a shift, and stayed –it was good news for all of us. No one was floating tonight. Hooray!

Recently, on returning to PedsICU after floating to a basic pediatric floor, a PICU nurse announced, "Man, is it ever scary on those basic floors? I'm never going to work there again –never again." We listened. What could be so terrible on a pediatric floor? It wasn't as though she had been caring for adults.

"Those basic kids actually walk around!" she announced. Walking pediatric patients was scary to a PICU nurse, whose perfect patient was sedated, paralyzed, intubated –and stable! But nurses had to take turns floating to other floors. A careful record was kept by the Charge Nurses as to who was next to float, and there had to be no errors in that list, or someone would want to know the reason why!

Some PICU nurses were resistant to working in the Rat Lab —AKA the Neonatal Intensive Care Unit, preferring instead to take their chances and float to a basic pediatric floor where the patients would likely be walking, talking, and probably crying. However, for most of us, the worst option was to work on a big-people floor.

"Big bodies, big medicines, and big poops. No way. I'm not going. I'm out of my comfort zone," was the rationale PICU nurses voiced to legally refuse to float to an adult floor. If it was *so* far out of her comfort zone, and clinical competence skill-set that she might make an error, she could refuse to go to a floor.

PICU nurses also believe, sometimes subconsciously, that some big people have themselves to blame for being hospitalized. That can happen, but some big people, like our kids, were in the wrong place at the wrong time, and developed diseases beyond their control.

***

At that moment Ellen breezed into the Nurses Lounge. Friendly, and in command, she was one of two regular night shift Charge Nurses. She meant business, especially at this moment of the shift. It was crunch time. Had everyone turned up who was scheduled? Had those who called in sick earlier, been crossed off the staffing list and been replaced? Ellen looked around the room and, seeing no strange faces, she sat down and relaxed.

"Good evening everyone ... thanks for coming to work...it looks like we have our full complement of staff," she announced. She was confident that the shift would go well, or at least start off well.

Ellen was one of the Night Charge Nurses who had been, by all accounts, the original Night Charge Nurse in the tiny PICU over the street, centuries before Noah and the Flood! The mother of sons, a daughter and grandkids, she had felt a mother's loss close up. Recently, one of her kids had died in an accident. It was painful seeing her bravely struggle with her loss, and when she returned to work, she had to face families in crises that were reminders of the fresh wounds in her soul. But over time, Ellen again proved herself to be the fearless leader we knew her to be.

Today, she was like a mother hen, and we were her little chicks. Ellen was a good, caring mother hen —even if a bit forgetful about who had requested what night off, when.

"I can't change my wedding date, Ellen," Mandy said. "It's all planned, and the invitations are out."

"Oh, my word, Mandy! You must have your wedding night off! I can't believe I did that." Mandy could believe it. We could all believe it. And so, the schedule was changed —again. Dear Ellen. With her numbers right tonight, she stood up to get our attention, and declared that no one would be floating as there had been another transport call.

"Right on, Ellen!" someone said.

"Our census is a little down," she continued, "but," she paused for effect, "there's been a *bad* MVA in Barstow. A roll-over," she said emphasizing the word *bad,* knowing that it held special significance to the crew. "The Transport Team flew —they left a while ago."

More cheers. *How sick can we be?* The Team flying, meant that the kid, or maybe kids, were definitely critically ill! This was good news! Two bad admits during the day, and more to come.

"We're on a roll."

"No floating for a while!"

"Cool."

The scenario was a sad reflection on how some minds work. Rational human beings would have been overwhelmed by such terrible situations —accidents, injured kids, ruined lives, near fatalities, cars totalled, and so on. Absolutely terrible. But somehow, PICU nurses had a different interpretation of the news.

Transporting critical kids? Cool.

What? Very critically ill kids? Wow...extra cool.

After a short prayer, we left the room, up-beat and chatting quietly with assignment cards in hand. The roll-over family needed prayer, and we sure wanted prayer! It was time to start our shift.

* * *

The Hospital Nursing Supervisor, the Supe, visited the ICUs within the first hour of the shift to check on their bed situations, and get a report from the Charge Nurse as to how the unit was running. At times, they called, but a personal visit was greatly appreciated. She, or he, in turn, gave the Charge Nurse an update on the state of the Peds ER, and any traffic accidents on the radar.

"Ellen, there are no kids in the ER right now, and the Barstow MVA," the Supe paused strategically, "I'm sorry, there were no kids on board after all. False alarm."

A handful of nurses had gathered to hear Brett's update. They stared blankly at him. Mumblings broke out about wasting time preparing rooms at the beginning of the shift when there was so much else to do. Why hadn't he let them know earlier?

Despite his poor health at times, quiet, efficient Brett was a favorite Night Supervisor, and knew precisely what to say to set Ellen, and her staff, on edge. He quietly turned to walk down the hall towards the double doors, as they watched in disbelief. Then, turning around with a smile on his face he said, "It's a joke. I can't lie."

The tension evaporated. "Get out of here, Brett, before I…" Connie, the secretary yelled, as the doors slammed behind him.

Ten minutes later the Transport Team called the floor, confirming the severity of the trauma. It wasn't funny. The kid was bad –but there was only one kid.

"They're taking off in 5-minutes, and will be landing on the pad in about 50-minutes," Ellen relayed. "They are going through Peds ER on their way here."

If the staff had been thinking more clearly when Brett dropped his bombshell, they would have known that a kid was coming –it was Ellen's first night on of a stretch of four. History clearly showed that when Ellen was in charge, it would be a busy night. Expecting a quiet one was out of the question. The words *Ellen* and *Quiet Night* were totally incompatible. Rarely, if ever, was it a quiet night when she was working, and tonight would be no exception.

It was usual to see her pushing beds from one end of the unit to another in the dead of night, or steering IV poles with one hand, with an extra med-infusion IV pump tucked tightly under her arm, while her free hand dragged a crib behind her. Only Ellen could routinely turn a pleasant, quiet night into a busy night, and busy shifts into hell in a handbasket! Rumor had it, that if PedsICU wasn't busy when Ellen came to work, she would flag traffic down outside the hospital, and direct every critical and moribund child through the Peds ER, and up to the floor, to make the unit "normal." That was a joke —or was it?

It was also true that Ellen transferred patients off the floor early in the shift to other pediatric floors, to make space for late-night admissions. This meant waking up umpteen day-shift nurses in case they wanted to come in early to work an 18-hour shift! It was hard to imagine that any Day Shift Nurses were lying awake, hoping, and praying, that they would be called in to work at 2 AM. The trick to getting nurses in early was to ask them before they left work the evening before, or have the secretary call Day Shift Nurses who were likely to come in extra early, before they got into bed. This scheme usually worked, but to guarantee any degree of success, it had to be tackled as soon as the night shift began.

One crisis that hit Ellen regularly was her ability to lose her paper brains, the detailed Shift Report on which she noted the specifics of all the patients on the floor. In the quiet of the night, the familiar *ding-dong* of the intercom sounded.

"If anyone finds my brains, please return them to me."

The usual titter of laughter followed this remark, but we all knew how difficult it was to survive a shift without our original report sheet, and all the more so, when it contained the particulars on up to 25-patients. With the lost Shift Report found, "Come and get it," reverberated around the floor, or the nurse trekked to the front of the unit, and dropped it off for her.

Corinne, one of the day shift Charge Nurses organized her crew like a friendly drill sergeant, and appeared to have the opposite effect from Ellen on the PICU bed census. This upset the night crew because Corinne emptied the beds during the day shift as fast as Ellen had filled them during the previous night. This meant that if they team-tagged, the night shift nurses admitted patients in droves, only to find the beds empty when they came back to work the next evening. Then they would admit like crazy again! Most nurses are specialist team-players, but not always on the same team!

***

An essential component of admitting a pediatric patient is to weigh the patient accurately as physicians prescribe all medications according to the little patient's weight. Electronic bed scales are a godsend, however, using sling scales or baby scales while lifting ventilator and IV tubing, catheters, drainage bag and cables off the scale to ensure accuracy, becomes a team effort, and a learned skill, especially if the child is very ill.

"Now write the weight down," is sage advice, for no nurse wants to put her colleagues through another weighing fiasco because she forgot the actual weight! *Duh!* Daily weights are usual, especially on kids who are retaining a lot of fluid, or who are less than a year old.

Another important aspect of admission is a thorough, extensive clinical assessment, and an immediate, acute stabilization of the patient. We ask parents to wait for the physician and nurse to complete their initial assessments, and settle the patient, before they can enter the unit to see their kid. For some kids, that might take minutes, while for others it can take much longer. These initial steps in caring for the child are important, and being able to work as a team, uninterrupted, for a short while, is very helpful for us – and the patient. Ultimately, it benefits the parents too. But the acute stabilization of a child in a critical condition takes more time than any frantic parent would expect. But there is no clear-cut answer as to how long parents should wait to enter the unit, and nurses differ in this matter, with some being more lenient than others.

"Let them in, now," Mia would always say. She had been a parent on the other side of the door, so she had her patient's parents at the bedside as soon as it was humanly possible, whereas –you guessed it, I was a little slower! Later on, the obnoxious parents who manipulate the system and are non-compliant with other requests, have to wait longer than do the polite, understanding parents who try to work with the policies, the nurses and the physicians. However, that first time, when their child rolls onto the floor, we do our best to get at least one parent promptly to the bedside.

* * *

We have good team players in PedsICU, not because our patients are huge and we need someone to physically help us –although some are large, but because ICU is a very pressure-filled environment and emergencies happen often. Nurses who fail to pull their weight, or who demand more of others than themselves, are recognized quickly. The nurse who requests help to lift a 4 kg child, or who frequently finagles getting the best assignment, or who asks others to hike to the front of the unit to get something for her, or him, is soon recognized. Teamwork is essential and nurses who repeatedly abuse their colleagues' kindness are looked upon as un-welcome extra baggage, and various tactics are implemented to get the message across to a lazy colleague.

"Sorry, I can't help. I am busy myself."

"No time at the moment. I am already late with an antibiotic."

"Sorry, I didn't know you wanted me to pick up your meds as well."

"I can help in a while but…"

Bold nurses may be even more direct with the spongers. "No way…just get your butt off that chair, and do it yourself!"

For the most part, this is not a problem as we are usually team players, and givers rather than takers. However, a chronic situation will crop up every-so-often, and with only two shifts per 24-hours, what goes around, comes around. An untidy nurse, who leaves their rooms a mess, may find it that way when they return 12-hours later. That negligence back-fires if the lazy nurse calls in sick, or chooses a different list. Then, an unsuspecting, on-coming nurse pays the price for the former nurse's laziness. However, the day of reckoning eventually comes.

Annual evaluations roll around –annually, and input is required from both Charge Nurses on the shift, and four colleagues. A lazy nurse will be hard pushed to find two nurses on their shift who are kindly disposed towards them, let alone two nurses on the opposite shift. It might just be time to declare war on their slovenly colleague!

It's no secret that nurses talk –and complain to one another about offending individuals and situations. It's a human characteristic. But writing the bare truth about a slovenly colleague on the official, annual evaluation, is difficult. Some nurses can't bring themselves to write the facts, choosing to ignore the reality. Others write about the problem obliquely, not wanting to acknowledge the harsh truth. They mentally question whether it will help their co-worker change into an appreciated team member. Are they doing their colleagues a service?

The reality is that following a lazy nurse means one has to spend valuable time bringing order to the kid's room, while still performing the routine cares for the patient. That extra work could include returning additional equipment, restocking drawers and cupboards, and getting hold of medicines that should have been ordered by the slothful colleague, but weren't. It gets old quickly.

Tony was a nurse in this order, or disorder, who worked the day shift. Some of the night staff regularly checked the assignment board on entering the unit to see where Tony had been working, so that they would avoid following his sloppy practices.

Fed up with the chaos that followed him, June, a Night Nurse, decided to take the matter into her own hands. Hoping to get the message over to him that she had had enough, she left one 3-ml syringe, one 10-ml syringe, one alcohol wipe, one Band-Aid, one Size 18 needle, one washcloth and one sheet in the room, when she went home in the morning. These were obviously very inadequate supplies for a 12-hour shift!

"It's time he got a taste of his own medicine!" June said as she left.

"You didn't!" Stacia gasped in disbelief. Stacia was a quiet Filipino nurse. "He's going to be unhappy."

"That's the whole point, Stacia. He should be unhappy, extremely unhappy."

"I bet he won't notice," I quipped.

This scenario caused more than a few chuckles — but sadly did not change the offending behavior! Tony remained the most inconsiderate, lazy nurse on the unit. Day, and Night Nurses repeatedly reported his lack of team spirit, and his slothfulness, to the Charge Nurses. It was common knowledge, and yet he kept turning up for work, and doing less than expected. That was until he was fired on the spot for something entirely unrelated. We didn't feel bad for him, in fact, the unit was mildly elated. He got what he deserved –finally!

TEAM PLAYERS'

Be warned. PICU nurses are team players, and if you aren't a team player, you won't be on the team very long!

CHAPTER 4

Chillin'

THE MICROCOSM OF THE PICU has its own stories -and skeletons in the cupboards. With a staff of around 80-nurses covering both shifts, friendships develop that make coming to work a time of reconnection. I was sure to learn something new, about somebody, during each shift.

With so many nurses, we were not at a loss for our own personal drama series. The excitement of engagements and weddings kept us mesmerized for a while, as did the anticipation of babies (and grand-babies), especially after infertility problems. Sometimes we chose to work in different areas of the floor to avoid pain, or joy, as we journeyed though our challenges. The trauma of a divorce, may be followed by a new relationship. We felt genuine happiness for a colleague who had survived a painful split, and then found true love again. How we hoped it would be a lasting, happy relationship.

Nurses with similar interests could always find others with that penchant, and social groups developed, most of which overlapped, and none of which were exclusive. The scrap-bookers brought in their new equipment, talked about scrapbooking fairs, and oooh-ed and aaah-ed at incredibly beautiful, manicured, album pages. The churchgoers spoke of their church picnics, and invited everyone to Christmas plays and special activities, Bibles studies and regular church services. The parents of school kids talked about the problems of car-pooling, of extra-curricular team sports schedules and the wonders of their incredibly talented children who won academic awards, were state champions in basketball, had won the local Spelling Bee, or played the leading role in a local community theater. Oh yes, we had amazing children! But what could you expect from such incredible nurses? If the exaggerations were too upsetting, we could drop out of that club and join another, or start a new one. We were social beings.

The biking enthusiasts talked of bikes, brakes, saddles, bike trails and the local biking club activities, upcoming races and their times, while the runners formed another lose group. We didn't run together, but we all ran and spoke the runner's lingo. We talked about running shoes, PBs, hitting the wall (or not hitting the wall), "goody" bags, race times, courses, ratings and the race bling we won. I wasn't the star of the group by any means, but I was out running marathons, halfs, and 10Ks –and not disgracing myself. Kai won marathons, so we all looked like losers compared to him –but when he became a veteran athlete, he too became mortal, settling for slower times.

The first Sunday in March, I walked onto the floor with an LA Marathon medal swinging from around my neck. Nothing special –everyone got a medal when they completed, or survived the race. "You didn't run today did you, Tabitha?" Connie asked as I shuffled past her desk.

"Yes," I replied. "Can't you see I'm hobbling?"

She couldn't, but my legs were a little tired. All I wanted was a quiet night – so that they could seize-up slowly, and avoid being a complete cripple for the next two days! My wish was granted. It was a quiet night, and I slept very well the next day.

Those less into sport were the shoppers, who hit the stores, often together, elated by steals they snatched from an unsuspecting bargain-hunter. The Disneyland crew chatted about the latest Disney gimmick that they just had to get on the day it came out –or the newest ride, or whatever the Disneyland crew talked about. It was as unknown to me as was the Vegas' group chatter. They carefully scheduled their time off to spend three days, for the price of two, in Vegas, and do the casinos and whatever. It was said that some had more fun on the buses going to and from Vegas, than at the casinos. It cost less too.

Regretfully, I was part of the 40s-club. We were no longer young chicks, but mildly seasoned and anticipating our journey towards an empty-nest, mounting college expenses and eventually graduating into the 50s club with a memorable over-the-hill celebration. We wondered what could be exciting at such an advanced age! Little did I realize I would still be working in the PedsICU when I was over the proverbial hill, along with other excellent "mature" nurses.

Working 12-hour shifts alongside one or two colleagues, gave us the occasional opportunity to talk about life, to provide support to one another and even a shoulder to cry on. The broad age range meant some staff had kids graduating from diapers, or kindergarten, while others were talking about high school graduations and proms.

Some of us were back in school completing graduate studies hoping that, in another year or two, we would be graduating with a coveted advanced degree. It was wishful-thinking to imagine that we would have spare time at work in which to study, but we often dutifully brought with us a text book which usually went home with us, un-read.

Eventually I graduated and when my name was called out at my graduation, my kids yelled loudly as they let go of helium balloons that floated towards the auditorium ceiling carrying a banner saying, "Go Dr. Mum" as I walked forward to receive my degree. Two of my doctoral committee waited to hood me and no doubt, when I bent down for the hooding, they were surprised to see a Union Jack carefully glued to the top of my mortarboard. Today, many students put messages on their graduation cap –but that is now.

Later that day, at a restaurant, my kids were on their best behavior as PICU nurses, friends from church, a few family members and my husband, sat around five tables to celebrate my finally completing a doctorate. It was a high day for me, after an exceedingly long slog through seemingly interminable studies, research and a dissertation. Surely no one had taken as long as I had? But finally, I had a doctoral degree and was elated.

After our meal, I stood up among a flotilla of helium balloons clinging to the ceiling, to thank my friends. It was the usual stuff. "Thank you for your support…I couldn't have survived without your friendship…This is one of the most memorable days of my life… Thank you, everyone…First and foremost, praise God... Yada-yada." But I meant every word I said – and had to sit down before I started to cry.

And so the ups-and-downs of PedsICU pass us by, sometimes from a distance, sometimes as a very close shave, and sometimes we are the target. And that was why *Night Light* survived for a while. Emergency surgeries, the death of a family member, the celebration of a new life – whatever, we were ready. Our ever-alert antennae picked up the unspoken distress of our colleagues who had unwittingly unloaded onto us more than they had meant to, or more than we wanted to hear. However, the support that we gave each other, sometimes carried us safely through some of the worst nightmares of our lives, be it the death of a child, the dissolution of a marriage, or another crisis. The small committee of a secretary, a leader, and a treasurer kept *Night Light* going. However, eventually, no one was willing to take over the volunteer positions. We all had busy lives, and taking on extra responsibilities became a burden. *Night Light* folded, leaving us once again to care for our friends in stressful, sad times, ad-hoc, and to hopefully celebrate with them in their joyful spells, perhaps somehow organizing a celebratory pot-luck for them. For me though, it was a sad end to an era –but life went on.

Most of the time, PICU nurses enjoy their work, although there are rough patches. Thankfully, these don't last. However, it is in those sad, bad times that a PICU nurse will ask, "Why am I working here? It is much too sad, and much too stressful."

And one nurse will reply, "We do it for the kids." And the crisis passes.

* * *

Accidents and illnesses happen in PedsICU nurses' homes, but may only afford a quick comment, and some practical advice.

"A headache? That's what Tylenol® is for. How many kilograms do you now weigh?" a nurse may ask her own child.

"It's too bad you scraped your knee… let me scrub the road rash clean… now, hold the dressing tightly… okay. Can you walk? You can? Right, go out to play."

"Oh, so you hit your head and lost consciousness for a few seconds. That's too bad. NPO for you. I guess

CHILLIN'

you won't be eating supper tonight after all. I'll keep an eye on you, just in case."

"You jumped off the carport, did you? Hmm...no wonder your leg hurts. I remember when ..." at which time the PICU-nurse-cum-mother launches into a story about ill-fated children who lost a leg or arm, or had a severe concussion. Those unfortunate children had holes drilled into their heads to measure ventricular pressure, "and if you want to know where your ventricles are, ask me later. I'm getting ready for work!"

Our children receive the inevitable safety lectures, but in time they tune us out. However, they having a PICU nurse for a parent, might save their lives, or someone else's. Our kids benefit from growing up with a knowledge of medical matters which they learn though osmosis. They are better able to deal with minor medical emergencies with aplomb at play or at school, and even later as adults. Most PICU nurses are safety conscious, and regularly issue commands to their young kids to reduce their risk of severe injuries, or to avoid fatal accidents.

"Wear your helmet."

"Don't swim alone."

"Wear your elbow pads, guys."

"Buckle up."

"Don't run with your mouth full."

"Look both ways, first."

Consequently, PICU parents are not the first ones to rush their children to the Peds ER, or demand a CT for stomach ache. We carefully perform routine pre-admission evaluations, and treat our kids as would any caring, knowledgeable parent before we take our kid to visit the pediatrician, or ER if we absolutely have to. Sadly though, occasionally PICU nurses' kids do end up in the PedsICU.

* * *

Most nurses have very big hearts hidden under their professional exterior of down-to-earthiness, and thrive on helping others. They are kind people, but this may be exploited by family members, demanding children or lazy husbands.

But kids and spouses, no longer only say "Aw, Mom, all the kids have Nikes®. I want a pair." Single, sought-after products expand exponentially to include the latest teen fashions, electronics, communication devices, I-phones, games, costumes for dance, sport and fashion shows, computers and software, vacations, and tools etc. The list goes on relentlessly, placing pressure on nurses earning "the big bucks" to cough-up, and pay for whatever their family *wants*.

A hard-working nurse might respond with, "Okay, honey. I'll work an extra shift this week to pay for your school trip," and go on to say, "I'll will buy the Nikes® for you this once …get you the I-phone 7 (or whatever is the latest model) …buy you a car…pay your/our/their car insurance…take you to Las Vegas for a weekend… pay for my mother's medications…pay my brother's bail," and so on. It can snowball into a never-ending begging routine – until the earner, worn out with extra shifts, firmly puts her, or his, foot down.

* * *

Some PICU nurses choose not to look after kids the age of their children, while others are the exact opposite.

They want to look after kids their children's age because they relate well to them, however, when some nurses become first-time parents, working in the PICU becomes an entirely different ball game. One day the rumor-mill started churning. Was it a joke, or for real?

Soon after the birth of her first child, Marilyn, a PedsICU nurse returned to work, only to find that everything was different now that she was a mother. She wasn't happy in PedsICU and submitted a written request to the Nurse Manager, asking her to exempt her from caring for kids who were likely to die. Sarah aired the subject during a break.

"You're joking," Stacia said in disbelief. Stacia was often unsure of when a joke was a joke —and when it wasn't.

"No," Sarah exclaimed, "it isn't a joke, Stacia. She wrote it —really."

"Give me a break," I exclaimed. "Why on earth is she working here if she doesn't want to work with kids who die? That's part of being a PICU nurse. It is, after all, a Pediatric...Intensive...Care...Unit. It's not a day nursery where all hell breaks loose when one child stubs his toe, or is hospitalized!"

We laughed. It was indeed a bizarre request.

"Well," Sarah said, "there's no way she will get Donna to agree to that. Marilyn's going to have to quit if she won't work with kids that *might* die."

And Marilyn did quit. Three weeks later she moved on to safer pastures where death wasn't continually knocking on the door. Donna could not accommodate Marilyn's request, and in her new role of being a mother, Marilyn had learned that caring for dying kids came too close to home for comfort.

* * *

It was shortly before Christmas, and Station One was bustling. The door-bell was chiming, phones were ringing and the secretary was multi-tasking, connecting the Attending with an in-coming transport call while organizing the next Transport Team to be sent out.

Ellen had completed the routine Charge Nurse activities of re-calibrating equipment, checking the Stat Carts on all five stations, updating patient data, confirming and entering diagnoses or changing the status on patients already on the floor. She had assisted her busiest nurses at the start of another crazy shift and was looking for some down-time.

It was 2 AM and a stack of stapled, up-dated report sheets was ready for the Residents and other staff to grab as they rushed by in the morning. She was so ready to chill.

Connie wore her usual late-night attire of a blue surgical gown wrapped around her 1 ½ times, and shoe covers over thick socks. She was not going to be cold tonight, and if she was, she would drape around her shoulders warm bath blankets from the blanket warmer, to complete her nifty outfit. She propped her feet up on the desk. Her shoes lay untidily underneath. She was ready to join any interesting conversation that drifted through the unit. If it wasn't interesting to begin with, it would be, for sue, by the time she had chimed in.

Ellen sat on a revolving chair, near the whiteboard that listed the rooms, the nurses' names and their occupants' last name. It was out of sight to visitors, but easily seen by the nursing and medical staff.

CHILLIN'

It was chill time.

Unusual for me, but very welcome, was the fact that time was dragging on Station One. Both my patients were on the road to recovery. One child was an 8-year-old asthmatic who would be transferred to the Step-down ICU in the morning, if everything went as planned. This little frequent-flier knew the hospital routines, and did not require much attention during the night as she slept most of the time. The monitor's clicking-sounds did not upset her, and she was a pro when it came to two-hourly vital signs. Four-hourly breathing treatments by the RT, did not faze her either. She was A-Okay. All I had to do was give her a few meds, and keep her IV going. Simple.

My other child was two months old, and admitted with febrile seizures. He would be staying on the unit for at least two more days, and had already been bathed and weighed. He was bottle fed every four hours, and slept most of the time. His monitors were set to catch any apneic, or bradycardic spells, so that I could intervene immediately. Amazingly, I was up-to-date with my charting, and time was dragging.

"Ross was in the ER yesterday," I calmly announced to Connie and Ellen who were sitting about 10-feet away from me. "He broke his arm."

That titbit of information caught their attention. Ross was my 18-year-old son. Connie sat straight up in her seat, "Well go on. Tell us what happened."

"He only fell off the roof," I answered.

"Only? Only fell off the what?" Connie exploded. "Do you mean to say you had him up on the roof for some sort of punishment, and he fell? Come on, Tabitha, even you wouldn't be as mean as that would you?"

I defended myself.

"Well actually, Connie," I started, "he was putting up Christmas lights, when he fell. That's all. It's was as simple as that."

"Oh, yes, Tabitha," she butted in, "that's all. Everyone falls off the roof putting up Christmas lights. It was as simple as that."

"Well, let me be absolutely accurate. He fell off the roof on Friday, and told me he was okay."

CHILLIN'

"I bet he said he was okay, with you being his mother!" she chided.

I reassured my listeners, "When he fell off the ladder, he grabbed onto the eaves, and a part of the eaves came away in his hand. Then he fell backward onto the grass. He didn't fall very far."

"Not very far," Connie burst out, "—but far enough to break his arm!"

Ellen listened.

"I wasn't there when it happened on Friday," I said, getting annoyed. "He was bundled up with ice packs by the time I came home later that day. I asked him the usual CMS questions, and I checked his radial pulses too."

I paused, knowing that my assessment was too cursory.

"I bet he daren't do anything else, Tabitha, with you as his mother! He knew you would have told him to toughen up," Connie said. "He knew his lines, poor boy, he knew better than to complain."

"And, as I said before I was so rudely interrupted," I continued, "I asked him if he was okay, and he said yes. So, I told him to take some painkillers and rest the arm, and I'd take a look at his arm when I got home in the morning —which was this morning. Well, yesterday morning —it's 2 AM now. I took one look at it while he was still in bed. He said he hadn't slept a wink all night, and that the pain was bad. I guess I then got a little wild-eyed," I said, and Connie gave Ellen a knowing look.

"Here it comes," Connie said, rolling her eyes.

"So I said to Ross, 'What do you mean you didn't sleep? Did you take any painkillers?'"

"I can just hear you," interjected Connie. "Bossy nurse ... the poor thing. In pain and you're complaining at him? Have you no sympathy?"

I thought for a moment. "Well, if I didn't when I went into his room, I sure did a moment later. I asked him to put his arm out for me to look at it, and when he unwrapped it, anyone could see he'd broken it! No wonder he hadn't slept." I paused. "I know I should have checked his arm myself before I went to work, but he said it wasn't painful, and he could move his fingers —so

CHILLIN'

I didn't. Anyhow, that is how he came to be in the ER Saturday morning. And now he has a cast on, and he's taking painkillers every four hours. He's doing much better," I added with a laugh.

"I'm glad he's doing okay now. Who would want a PICU nurse for a mother?" Ellen replied sympathetically. She hesitated one moment, and then continued. "I know exactly what you mean."

Connie had a nose like a bloodhound for stories, and knew that something else was about to unravel. "Don't tell me you are as bad as Tabitha, Ellen?" she said in disbelief. "Why, your poor kids!"

"Yes, I think I was worse than Tabitha. My youngest came in after a soccer game one night, and said that his leg was in terrible pain. You know how it is —16-year-olds fooling around and wasting time as they do? Well, I told him to take it easy that evening, and it would get better."

"Oh no, Ellen," Connie jumped up in anticipation of another tragedy. "He hadn't broken his leg, had he?" she guffawed.

"Well, actually –yes," Ellen said.

Connie laughed out loud. It was too much. How could two PICU nurses have kids fracturing two extremities, without their mothers knowing it? It was too funny!

"I told him to stay on the sofa that night, if he really couldn't make it up the stairs —which he couldn't, of course. I left him watching TV, and went to bed."

Connie, anxious to get every last ounce out of the story, interjected. "You didn't do that really did you, Ellen?"

"Yes, I did. When I came down in the morning, I realized that he had broken his leg, and we went off to the ER."

Ellen smiled. At least she and Tabitha couldn't be accused of panicking! Quite the opposite.

And the night wore on.

The stories illustrated that PICU nurses' children sometimes had to complain very loudly, in the hopes that a severe injury would elicit an adequate response! Perhaps nurses' kids didn't have the advantages that one might think they had at first –but telling stories, true ones, surely made a few slow hours pass more quickly.

* * *

I pulled myself out of my seat and ambled over to Room 2 where the two-monther was sleeping soundly. I checked the clock. It was almost time for vital signs and another feed.

The bottle of formula bobbed in a container of hot water. I documented his vital signs on a paper towel, gave the baby his meds and threw the used, oral syringe across the room, into the trash can that was under the window, scoring a basket. Wrapping the baby into a tidy cocoon of blankets and cables, I sat down carefully in the bare wooden rocker.

He is a cute little thing, I thought as he hungrily chugged down 120 ml of formula, burped and went to sleep in my arms. Easing myself out of the chair, and keeping the baby bundled and connected to the monitors, I gently laid him in the crib.

The day shift would be arriving soon. Through the window, the dazzling snow-capped peak to the north side emerged from inky-blue darkness, like a silver pyramid. Within minutes the sky morphed into a rich crimson color. I turned to the computer, entered the vital signs and Is & Os. It would be another beautiful winter's day, and best of all, soon it would be time to go home.

The murmur of PICU's day shift nurses swinging through the doors winged through the airways. The smell of fresh coffee crept around the corners as they piled into the Nurses Lounge, ready for another shift. They had their own stories, their own skeletons. We passed each other twice a shift –at the beginning and at the end of our shifts –then we went our separate ways. They were a different crew, with different stories, but still our colleagues, and members of the PedsICU team of nurses, and we cared about each other.

CHAPTER 5

Surrogates

IT WOULD BE SIMPLISTIC to state that PICU nurses are only professional monitor-watchers, IV-hangers, and vital sign takers for very critically ill kids. All nurses are care-givers, but PICU nurses' charges are vulnerable, they are young, and usually they haven't yet learned how to control their immediate environment. Nurses take on a variety of surrogate roles. This may depend on how confident they are in their role as an adult in general, and especially in a kid's world, and on how broad a view they have of nursing and caring for their patients. This determines whether they are willing to step into the breach to protect their charges emotionally, and physically (if needs be) at work, and whether or not that role extends to outside the workplace in public, where they might be on their own, and vulnerable. Will they speak up when they see a neglected child? Will they speak up, when they have a hunch that a child's home-life is not quite right? Will they take action, or leave it to someone else? Not all PICU nurses are ready to take these types of matters into hand away from the safety of the workplace, but are confident in their role as adult and nurse, in the workplace.

* * *

My three children were middle school-age kids when we drove up to the grocery store in an out-of-the-way part of town. As I rolled into the parking lot, my eyes were drawn to three kids, about the same age as my children, on bicycles, and not wearing helmets. They had probably gone into the store, but when I saw them, they were getting on their bikes to pedal off down the street. My eldest son knew what was going to happen.

Immediately he said, "No, Mum, no," as he slid down on the front seat, out of sight to the kids.

It took a matter of seconds for the story to unravel. By now, my younger kids were lying low in the back seat. "Don't say anything, Mum," my eldest admonished. But it was too late.

Pulling up beside the kids, I rolled down my window. "You know guys, it is dangerous to ride your bikes around the streets without wearing a helmet –and against the law." Taken aback, they looked at me for a few seconds.

"Head injuries are something you don't want to experience," I said, "–believe me." The boys were beginning to flee from the front of the store. "Please wear helmets…and be careful on your bikes. I don't want to meet you in the hospital!"

The kids were one their way as my children began to emerge from their hiding places. Did I make any difference? Probably not, but who is to know. Now with two adult children who are school teachers, they might look at this situation differently, but at that time, I was an embarrassment to them. So was my mother to me.

Aren't all mothers an embarrassment to their children at one time or another? That's normal.

Twenty years later, I had left work. It was around 7 PM and dark. The wind whipped through the parking lot. I was up north, and the temperature was well below freezing. Two parents were hauling two young kids out of their vehicle to go to the store. The parents wore jackets and long pants, and I was dressed in layers. But the youngest child was wearing no shoes and only a little tee-shirt and shorts. She was about a year old. *Shall I say something or not?* "Excuse me, ma'am. Your child needs more clothes on when the weather is so cold." That was as far as I got. Both parents turned on me with expletives and yelled at me, telling me to mind my own business, as they fled into the store. I am better prepared for the situation, should it happen again, but how far does one go to protect children from neglect, or abuse of any form? Is it my business? Is it your business?

There are no simple answers to these questions, but PICU nurses are often called to be stand-in parents, or surrogates for their charges, when someone is missing.

* * *

PICU kids often have to endure physical pain, and life becomes very scary for them, on our unit. Needles, white coats, closed doors, noisy equipment, rustling paper and blue towels. These can be scary when you are a kids and no one is with you. Sometimes parents are asked to step outside their kid's room for a procedure, and while a parent, or a substitute parent might be able to stay at the bedside, it is often left to the PICU nurse to step into the parent's shoes to keep their little kiddo happy. How miserably we fail.

Moises, a tough 9-year-old kid, was in that position. He needed a hand, a substitute hand, to hold. He was scared and alone. Moises had fractured his leg when scrubbing a jump on his dirt bike. Waking up after surgery in a strange hospital, Moises saw large metal pins protruding from either side of his leg. White gauze, soaked in a reddish-brown antiseptic ointment, partially covered the bolts protruding from his knee. Not knowing what they were, his heart rate increased considerably as he stared at what looked like huge, ugly, rusty metal bars leaking grungy, old blood.

Moises' fear persisted even though Heidi, a happy, upbeat nurse in her early thirties, gently bathed him, cleaning his abrasions and removing dust and grime. Not only was he embarrassed at being bathed by a stranger, but he became rigid with fear as he felt her wash his badly scraped arm. Ingrained gravel and dirt rolled around on his skin as she carefully bathed his road-rash. "I'm giving you extra pain medicine, Moises," Heidi said gently as she increased the IV analgesics again, but his frantic cries got louder, and his eyes grew as big as saucers, from fear and pain.

"Mommy, I want mommy. Mommy," he yelled, whipping his arm away from Heidi —but Mommy wasn't there, and once again he had to make do with Heidi.

From across the station, his cries brought back painful memories to me.

* * *

I changed into my scrubs, and after kissing each of my children good-bye, I made my way to the door. The youngest was then about 5-years-old, and started howling. She scrambled out of bed and ran across the kitchen floor in her pajamas, her little bare feet pattering across the cold tiles. "Don't go, Mummy," she screamed, "don't go!"

The noise aroused her brothers, who joined her in anguished tones, but thier daddy pulled her off my legs so that I could go to work. I shut the door behind me, knowing her daddy would be hugging her, however, even as I got into the car, I could still hear her crying, "Mummy, Mummy. Don't go Mummy." But I did, and with tears welling up, I drove off, intent on being a reliable member of the staff, professional and —cold. Couldn't I have given up one shift for them?

More than 10-years later, Moises' cries brought back the raw reminder of brushing off my kids to go to work.

* * *

At first, Moises didn't notice the support team Heidi had summoned to help her finish his bed bath and change his linen. Then, although he was covered and clean, his fear rose to another level when he saw three other nurses suddenly appear beside his bed.

"Moises, we're here to help you," said a nurse with a swinging pony-tail. He stared at her. "If we don't get you up the bed now, it won't get done until the next shift is here, and then they will have to pull you much further up the bed."

Moises looked at the four nurses beside his bed and swallowed hard. "Will it hurt?" he gulped. Telling the truth comes with being a PICU nurse. Even if it is not what a kid wants to hear, we always tell the truth —to some degree. It is only fair. "Yes, Moises, it will hurt," Heidi said gently, adding, "I am sorry. You've got extra pain medicine on board, but it will hurt. Hang tough. We'll be careful, and quick as possible. Then it'll be over." Moises panicked and began to cry.

I watched the scenario from my room. I thought of my kids begging and pleading for me to stay, not just that one time, but at other times too. I missed a few band performances too, and baseball games because of work, and had denied them a sleep-over or two. How did it make them feel? Had they thought that they were not as important as work to me? Had parenting become more complicated now that they were no longer little kids? Had I been a "missing" parent?

"No, no, don't move me," Moises yelled as the tears ran down his cheeks. "No. No."

But the nurses took their places beside his bed. One took the strain of the leg-weights hanging at the bottom of his bed, and two nurses held onto either side of the draw-sheet underneath him. They stood poised for action, waiting for the count.

"It's okay to cry Moises," Heidi said to him as she looked into his eyes. "We've got to do it Moises —but we'll be *real* careful. Here Moises, hold my hand," she said as she grabbed his hand. He held on. Then giving a one-two-three, they hauled him up the bed as he screamed at the top of his lungs and gripped Heidi's hand like a vice.

The three nurses left as quickly as they had come, leaving Heidi holding Moises' now limp hand in hers. She sat down beside him. "I'm sorry Moises. It must have hurt a lot...You did a great job... I'm so proud of you."

He took his hand out of hers and looked at her, "It hurt a lot."

I turned away and checked the monitor above my patient wondering what his life was like at home? What would he remember about being pulled up the bed, in another 10-years? Pain, fear, lack of control, aloneness, or his sweet nurse? But boys of Moises' age, and older, have an added struggle when it comes to crying —they don't want to cry. Crying is for little kids, not for them. It isn't cool to cry. But PICU nurses know that facing so many challenges may make it impossible *not* to cry —and that is okay.

Hey Peter, Jay, Kasey, Mikayla –it's okay to cry. We know it's scary here, but it is okay to cry…big kids cry … tough kids cry…it's normal to cry. The bottom line is that having a parent at the bedside is usually the most important thing for any kid when life is terrifying, like it can be in PedsICU.

* * *

The enclosed, long, hallway ran the length of the unit, from the front desk to the wall at the very end of the unit. It thwarted "looky-loos" from prying into kids' rooms. Once visitors got to a station though, they could meander past rooms getting an eyeful of a critically ill kid, whose family was probably going through a much worse time than they were. Some individuals could not conceal their curiosity, but stood stock-still, captivated by what they saw, staring at a very ill child. This situation gave the nearest nurse the unenviable task of getting the inquisitive visitor's attention, and making sure they moved along.

"Ma'am," I said, one day, to the young woman staring into Room 8. Nothing happened.

"Excuse me, ma'am," I said, a little louder. *There is no backing down now.* Sarah, my colleague, began to chart with enthusiasm with her head down. She feared what was going to happen. Pretending not to notice, she focused intently on the screen in front of her. *Still no response.* Now, determined to follow through, I was compelled to get up from my charting, and tap the mesmerized visitor on the arm.

"Er... ma'am, would you please move along? It is important for our kids to have privacy."

If all went well, the on-looker would apologize, and continue on her way, However, occasionally this type of request led to a retort such as, "You mind your own business, and I'll mind mine!" This made no sense to me, as it was clear that they weren't minding their own business! Had they been, I would not have started the conversation. But, even these individuals, would usually start moving towards the nearest exit, eventually. *Mission accomplished.* I had been an advocate for that patient's privacy –and I had applied the policy.

For nurses who do not like upsetting a patient's family –that is most of them, this situation is overlooked, and left for the next "mature" nurse to encounter. However, that mature nurse would have preferred that the problem had been addressed promptly, as per unit policies —and polite society! Dealing with this type of scenario is understandable, because nurses have enough problems dealing with their patients and their patients' families over a 12-hour shift, without voluntarily piling more aggravation on themselves. But who is going to stand up for a kid's privacy, if it isn't a nurse?

* * *

A trait we love to see in our patients' parents is reliability –as do their kids. Trustworthy parents develop that same trait in their child, plus reliability, and endurance, which are important components in resiliency, the attitude that helps children successfully face life's challenges. Children can endure almost anything if they can trust even one parent, but it is almost impossible to develop trust when parents lie to their kids. How can they trust their parents? Or us? It is impossible. And lying parents make matters a lot worse for a kid's nurse.

"Go to sleep, Honey," the parent says sitting quietly at the kid's bedside amid the clicking monitors under the timeless quivering, green, red and blue electronic rhythms that repeatedly rush across an otherwise black screen. Peace reigns. The child feels safe. Their Mommy or Daddy is right by their side. But…once they fall asleep, confident in their parent's presence, they get up and leave. Panic sets in when the child awakens, alone, with no parent in sight. In that first waking moment, confused and frightened, their world falls apart and the nurse has to left to pick up the fragments. She is a poor replacement for a kid's mother, or father, and is unlikely to have much time to spare in the PICU.

Arely can a nurse dally at a child's bedside, so the hunt for a substitute parent begins. Child Life Specialists (CLS) are on the short list. PICU is fortunate to have some excellent CLS on their team. CLSs are skilled at making kids feel secure and special when these kind, professional play therapy team members are available, but their scope of practice is extensive and busy with many activities. If available, they are in demand by patients who enjoy electronic games, X-boxes etc. or if they enjoy movies. Sometimes a CLS will even chill with a lonely little child and watch a movie with them, or help them color, paint or do a craft. CLSs have a magnificent arsenal of activities for all ages of children including toys, puzzle books, jigsaw puzzles, movies and much more for a lonely child.

But, for little kids, under two years old, a visit from a Snuggler might calm their jaded nerves and keep them content for a while. Snugglers are volunteers who undergo a full background check before being deemed safe to work with babies and little kids and are a phone-call away. Sadly, PICU has to share these angels with other little people on all the pediatric units, and especially with the NICU. Most Snugglers are women, but a few are men. Their sole job is to pick up and cuddle distressed infants and babies (under the nurse's supervision) or to play with them as a loving grand-parent would. Babies quickly settle when rocked, sung to or snuggled by a friendly, older person who has the knack of comforting distressed little kids.

"I love my job," said Noreen, a 74-year-old Snuggler. "The nurse is happy, the baby is happy, and I am blessed. What could be better?"

I know what's better —being snuggled by your mommy or daddy.

CHAPTER 6

Gown Up!

I RARELY CALLED IN SICK. I loved my work, had bills to pay and couldn't lie. Staffers would believe me if I said I had fallen off a rock-face or been eaten by a bear while hiking along a lonely trail, but not well? "You're never sick, Tabitha! Stay home, girl, it must be the bubonic plague if you're ill!"

My mother was a strong, tough woman, so perhaps it was partly genetics, and partly due to a healthy active lifestyle. But whatever it was, it paid off. I was rarely ill. That was even the case every winter when pneumonia and bronchiolitis hit the floor in a whirlwind. It could last for weeks, despite the weather being mild compared with the real winter experienced in northern states. Yellow isolation gowns, purple or blue disposable gloves, and pink or white masks became everyday attire to combat the spread of respiratory diseases throughout the unit. Also, cases of viral meningitis (for at least the first 24-hours after admission), bacterial meningitis, tuberculosis, and other contagious diseases, sent us running to find cover-gowns.

"If I have to put on another mask this shift," a nurse declared as I passed her room with my shift assignment in hand, "I will die!" I knew what she meant.

In the infectious season, isolation gowns were a priority. We made frantic phone calls to housekeeping for more yellow gowns and boxes of masks to be brought to our rooms to fill isolation cart drawers, as our supplies dwindled. Boxes of small, medium, large and extra-large gloves were stacked high on the top of carts, ready to cover any sized hand. And, at times, we hauled armloads of gowns out of secret stashes in anterooms, or

GOWN UP!

from hidden corners in the supply rooms. Despite our best efforts to avoid RSV each winter, most PICU nurses succumb to the infection (once) and then maintained immunity for the rest of the season, only to be hit by next year's variant 12-months later.

Some night staff, though, developed a strange affinity to clean coveralls. If they didn't find the superior quality, green or blue line gowns from the OR to wrap themselves in for the slow, night hours –that rarely occurred, they used yellow isolation gowns. Darryl, an affable, un-flappable PICU nurse felt undressed if he wasn't wearing a yellow gown. Consequently, when he left for a position in a neighboring city, we threw a farewell party for him and insisted that all party-goers wore spanking new, clean, yellow isolation gowns. No goobers on the sleeves or invisible viruses. *No siree! Spotless.* We were dressed appropriately for the occasion, ready for cake and ice-cream, laughter and even tears!

Once a nurse has peeled off the last gown and clingy mask for the shift, she knows exactly what she'll do when she's clocked out. "Shower time, folks. I can't wait!"

Not only am I healthy, but my children are too, and I am thankful. God has blessed us with good health, and yet the reality is that hospitals are filled with ill people, including kids. The simple lifestyle I experienced as a child, was partly because we had no car and no television, ate whole grain foods and were vegetarians. And no sweets (candy) were allowed. This lifestyle was weird by many people's standards, but my mother was bold, and I guess I blindly followed her example. I did not mind being thought of as peculiar. It was normal to me. In nursing school, I didn't quite fit in. I did not smoke, drink alcohol, party or take drugs —street drugs or prescribed medications, except for the occasional OTC pain-reliever, and did not pamper myself with luxuries. Swimming most days in the outdoor, unheated pool at the Nurses Home was free and fun, if a little bizarre, but stopped when it snowed. Just too much shock when I dived in. Bicycling 12-miles to visit my sister Rebecca at college, was a little crazy too, apparently —but kept me healthy in my student days.

It is possible to rationalize that the lifestyle choices adults have made, contribute to some of their hospitalizations, but not kids. Adults' health problems have finally caught up with them. That can be true with respect to lifestyle diseases, or, as some call them, Diseases of Choice, such as obesity, Type 2 diabetes and its complications, hypertension, COPD, coronary artery disease, lung cancer and some other cancers, and more. These diseases challenge my sympathy radar.

But kids are different. Why would God allow accidents to happen to them and for them to get injured in MVAs, or let them suffer the results of abuse, neurological deficits or genetic diseases? Life is not fair and I do not have good answers. My only response is that humanity is still dealing with sin, the result of Satan's choice to rise up against the leadership of God. The wages of sin is death -and what precedes it. The war between good or evil is still going on and critically ill kids are pawns in this battle. However, the Bible describes God as providing an eternal, perfect home in the future for the faithful and, in the meantime, it is my privilege to work with kids who are probably experiencing what they don't deserve.

***

It was early spring and recently Station Three had been called "Suction City," because most of the patients there were kids with respiratory illnesses. Some were frequent fliers who lived in a Pediatric Extended-care Facility a few miles from the hospital. As permanent residents at that facility, some were fragile and often came to the PedsICU. However, others had robust, resilient health which meant that they came to the PICU only when overwhelmed by an infection. All of the kids at this facility needed some respiratory support. Many had trachs and were on ventilators much of the time. With respiratory infections and thickening secretions, they surprised their caregivers by unexpectedly occluding their airway. This surprising turn of events required them to be rushed to the Peds ER and often up to the PedsICU for aggressive treatment including antibiotics, intravenous fluids, ventilatory support, and suctioning around the clock. A few days in PICU, and then on the Step-down ICU, usually pulled them through the episode, and they returned to the Extended-care Facility until another crisis hit. If these chronic little children were ever made a DNR, a total airway occlusion meant the end of a sad little life. I can imagine that God shed tears when He saw these little people's lives, and yet I don't understand it —but then I'm not God.

GOWN UP!

While some of these little people are somewhat endearing, others are anything but charming. Kevin was on Station Three in the corner room, paired with Lindsey, another severely developmentally delayed, and physically disabled child. Kevin had lived in the Children's Home for almost 7-years and was only marginally responsive, whereas Lindsey was 6-years-old and lived at home. She was lovingly cared for by her parents. Unlike many severely developmentally delayed kids, her family adored her. Lindsey smiled occasionally, recognized her parents and cried too. Lindsey's parents were caring and we admired their dedication to her. A little over 3-years before, Lindsey was paralyzed in an MVA. It was a tragedy. Now she was growing fast and putting on weight and had become a chunky little girl. And, if the truth be told, she was becoming rather too much for her family to handle any longer.

It was the beginning of another shift and I was in a good mood.

"I won the prize," I announced as I sat down next to Beth. "It'll be fun, fun, fun all night! Suction City here I come! Hand over the suction catheters, Beth! It's a hold-up!"

Beth was ready to oblige, and give me every suction catheter she could find (used and unused) and her report. She wanted to get out quickly. It had been a long day.

"Forty percent oxygen for Kevin, fifty for Lindsey. Suction hourly –or more often, G-tube-feedings every six hours for Kevin –every three hours for Lindsey: check residuals, bathe, weigh and G-tube-care, turn every two hours, antibiotics in the fridge and their meds are locked in their room. No visitors for Kevin today. Parents came to see Lindsey. Got it?"

"Yep," I said. "I bet that was the shortest report you have ever given, Beth. Now go and take a shower. You are beginning to smell like a goober yourself!"

Beth was glad to leave. Who wouldn't be? It had been a goobery day.

I quietened down and planned out my shift. Turns, feedings, baths, medications. On and on, round and round. It would be a seemingly, never-ending night, and the work was so futile, especially for Kevin. He would never be neurologically normal and never have a loving family to care for him. He was just Kevin, almost a nobody. This was Kevin's life. And Lindsey? Eventually, she would get too big for her family to care for her or complications would over-take her and time would march on without her being part of her family. She would probably end up like Kevin. Another unfortunate child that medical science kept alive, until it didn't.

I checked the isolation carts outside the rooms. Not enough gowns for the long shift ahead of me. "I'm going in search of gowns," I said to the nurses exchanging report at the station, and went off down the hall, returning a few minutes later with an armful of extra gowns which I divided, and shoved in both isolation carts, leaving a few stray sleeves hanging unceremoniously out of the stuffed drawers. I was ready for the shift. *Let it begin!*

"I sure am glad I didn't do my hair before I came to work," I mumbled as I struggled into the yellow paper gown and fought with the double, narrow, strong, rubber bands that had to be expanded under pressure, to secure the infamous N-95 masks in place. "How come we don't have any regular masks? Just my luck. These are an abomination." No one was listening. I hated these masks. And so the shift started.

At 11.30 PM I ripped off my gloves and balled up my gown and mask, and threw them into in the trash. Turning, I dropped a dollop of alcohol-based sanitizer gel into one hand and rubbed my hands together. My hair stuck to my forehead and the sides of my face as I emerged from Kevin's room. "I need a drink," I said expertly sliding Kevin's door shut with the back of my foot, and walked to the Nurses Station before slumping down in my chair. Betty and Karola looked up.

"What happened to you?" Betty asked.

"I haven't seen you for two hours," added Karola. "I thought you had suctioned yourself down the Yankauer with the biggest, slimiest goobers for sure —by accident of course!"

"Ha! Ha!" I said between gulps of water. "Very funny! And tell me pray, why didn't you look for me in the suction canister then?" They laughed.

After recovering a little, and swigging some more water, I announced, "I have just completed my 10 PM medications!"

"Congratulations, Tabitha!" Betty teased. "It is now 11.30 and your midnight meds are due in exactly 30-

minutes. We can trust you to be on time with your medications all the time —sure!"

"R-i-g-h-t," I said. "Earlier I thought I would impress you both by giving one kid his meds and G-tube feeding on time for a change –and bathe him too. I guess I was wrong. I went into Kevin's room long before his 10 PM feed when his meds were due. I just knew I would be in and out in a matter of minutes. Wrong. I stepped out to do Lindsey's vital signs —late again, and was back in with Kevin by 1030. I bathed him, weighed him and got him looking spotless, and started his feeding and then it went down-hill from there. Good grief, if he didn't start gagging and coughing!" Karola and Betty anticipated what happened next and began to smile. "The gravity-fed feeding flew up the syringe and shot out of the top, soaking my mask –and his clean bed!" My entertaining commentary was all Karola and Betty needed to set them off laughing. "Sure glad I had that horrible mask on," I added. They nodded sagely. "I tipped what was left of his feeding back into the graduate, and suctioned him. There was a goobery-mess everywhere. It was gross. His nose, his trach and then?" I looked up expectantly, "He did the largest poop ever! It oozed out around his diaper, and onto his newly changed bed!" I swiveled my chair and sucked down another gulp of water. "So, I started all over again…bathing and changing —but he didn't cough when I did his feed this time! Praise God. I don't think I could have sweated through another clean up again."

My audience knew full well how caring for two Suction City kids could challenge any nurse's skill, but this was too funny —to them. One and one-half-hours to do a bath, a weight and feed a kid? Whatever next? They roared with laughter forgetting it was almost midnight. "You forgot the cardinal rule, Tabitha. You should have fed and *then* changed him. Hellooo —anyone home?"

"And you should have called for help," Karola volunteered sympathetically.

"Yes –and called and called and called," I scolded. There was silence as I righted myself in the chair thinking I should look marginally professional. "I guess I should have known I could not win against two developmentally delayed kids. Solomon was right. Pride does go before a fall. I should have never thought I could get three things done on one kid on time. I am truly humbled."

It is incredible how such simple tasks can bring one down to earth with a bump! Suffice it to say, not only did I survive the shift, but Kevin and Lindsey looked bright-eyed and bushy-tailed at shift-change, when Beth returned.

"Same old," I said as she rolled out her report sheet. "But I learned a lesson tonight –and if you want to know what I learned, ask Karola or Betty. I am sure they would love to tell you their version." I picked up my backpack, and keeping it at arm's length, I slid into the hallway, "I'm off for a shower!"

CHAPTER 7

Changing Places

TONIGHT WILL BE MUCH SWEETER *for sure*, I thought as I almost skipped down the hall to Station Three. Tonight was the last of four shifts in a row, and there would be no more shenanigans with Kevin for me!

Lindsey was still in Room 14, but my list had been split, to spread the goobers around – figuratively speaking. I was not going to get upset about that –a PSIF kid couldn't be worse than Kevin. Or could it?

When the lists were assigned, I had to choose one of my kids from the previous night and add one more kid. It was a no-brainer. It was either Kevin with a new MVA kid, or Lindsey with a 12-year-old PSIF kid. "I'll take Lindsey," I nobly volunteered.

* * *

During school vacations, Pediatric Orthopedic Surgeons schedule surgeries with the expectation that there will be enough beds to accommodate their needs. That works for kids. They recover while school is out, and everyone is happy.

Spinal instrumentation surgeries are common vacation surgeries for teens. Rods are placed in the back to straighten it in cases of severe scoliosis. These kids are called PSIF kids, to avoid the mouthful of Posterior Spinal Instrumentation and Fixation. By the time the child is scheduled for surgery, they have often experienced significant back pain, have been unable to participate in sports at school and been the butt of cruel jokes. PSIF kids have one especially good thing going for them too. They gain 1 ½ - 2 inches in height as a result of the surgery. *Cool – very cool.*

CHANGING PLACES

The bad thing going for nurses caring for PSIF kids is that PSIF kids have a reputation for being spoilt kids. Over the months, or even years, many of them have manipulated their families to cater to their every desire, and become scheming wimps. Wimps are not sought-after patients, and while this isn't always the case, many nurses are not anxious to look after PSIF kids –just in case. So taking Lindsey with her goobers, and Emily with new rods in her back, was a risk, and I knew it.

There was one other nurse with me at the station, Mandy, a sweet-natured, cute young nurse who had recently married the love of her life. Mandy would be fun to work with for sure. It was Mandy's first night of three, and she had "lucked-out" with Kevin, and a new kid called John. The shift would be pretty routine for Kevin and Lindsey –suctioning, bathing, turning, suctioning (again), giving medicines, suctioning (once again), etc. Mandy and I would team up as necessary in caring for them, and our other two kids, as the need arose. It should be a regular night —whatever that meant. *No sweat.*

John's room was directly in front of the Nurses Station. He was in Room 13, a good room from the nurse's perspective as when she looked up from her computer, she could see directly into her patient's room. She did not have to crane her neck, or scoot her chair across the floor, to see her patient. John would be easily visible from the station. However, there was one problem. John wasn't visible because the curtains were drawn tightly across the glass-fronted room, leaving only a gap on the left through which his family, and Mandy, came and went. I could not see John. *Oh well... he's not my kid... but later on, I'll be covering for Mandy.* And I left it at that. As I planned my shift, I scanned the glass doors and windows of John's room, checking for a little pink, cut-out, laminated bear stuck somewhere on the glass indicating an imminent, or recent death. There was no bear. *What a relief.* But it was a little strange.

The night started with a bang. Emily had returned from surgery 10-minutes before report time and was situated in her bed by the day staff. She was very sleepy – fortunately. I had a long list of doctor's orders to take off the chart as soon as I was free, but Lindsey's vital signs and medications weren't due for half-an-hour. I scanned through the list of orders: change the IV, bring in the SCDs and get them operating, set up the PCA pump and instruct Emily (and her hovering parents) how it works

—and how not to use it. Get the antibiotics on board on time, turn her every two hours, and so on. Very routine.

As soon as possible, I set to on Emily's orders. I introduced myself to her parents, and to her, but she appeared to be out of it. Did she realize I was her nurse?

I programmed the PCA pump according to the physician's orders so that Emily could not overdose herself. During that first night, PSIF kids were often not alert enough to remember how to give themselves a dose of medicine, so patients might wake up, crippled with pain and screaming and, illegally, the parent provides the occasional shot of medication to keep the little pumpkin happy –which is not the purpose of Patient Controlled Analgesia! It was unlikely that a parent would overdose their child, but thankfully, by the following day, the kid usually had firm control of the PCA button.

"Okay Emily, listen up," I said clearly, to get through the mists of anesthesia. Emily opened heavy eyelids and gave me a blank stare. "Emily…listen up. I'm Tabitha, your nurse and now I'm going to tell you how to give yourself pain medication, and then you are going to do it for yourself. I know you have been through this before, but the anesthetic will wear off soon, and you will be in pain, so this little button is your friend." I held the clicker in front of Emily who struggled to stay awake. "When you start to get pain, press the clicker on the top —here," I said as I pointed to the button, "and press it with your thumb. It will give you a pre-programmed dose of pain killer... you can do this every 10-minutes...you can't overdose yourself as the medicine will make you drowsy, and when you are asleep, you won't be able to give yourself any medication."

No doubt Emily vaguely remembered being told about operating the PCA pump before surgery, but it was very confusing now. After repeating the directions, I gave Emily command of the button. "Okay, Emily...press the clicker on the top, and listen." A short peep sounded as Emily pushed the button. Later I documented that I had educated Emily on how to use the PCA pump. Turning to both of Emily's parents I added, "And please don't give Emily the medication yourself. We want her to control her pain," and I reviewed the purpose of the PCA pump for them.

Emily's parents, Elaine and Marcus, were very friendly and appreciated all that was being done for their daughter. Elaine sat beside the bed on the recliner, while

Marcus made phone calls off the unit, going back and forth as he wished. Emily had an older brother who had just graduated from high school. Emily's parents were proud of this fact, and I soon realized, by the conversation, that Emily was probably a loved, but pampered little sister and daughter.

"Elaine, what are you guys planning to do tonight? When will you be going home?" *Oops – that was a little in the face,* I thought. *But how else can I find out?*

"We are staying all night," Elaine answered. *Crap.* "We are going to stay with Emily for the next three days." *Whoa! Isn't that a little over the top?*

"I see," I gulped. *On second thoughts, that won't be so bad ... It might even work out well for me – and the rest of us. They're attentive parents, and things are going along well. And Emily? Well, she is the tiniest bit demanding and whiny...so perhaps her mom, staying at the bedside, will make everyone's life easier. Her mom will deal with Emily's complaints first.*

"I think that will work," I stammered. "But only one of you will be able to stay in the room during the night. I'm sorry. It's one of our rules."

"Don't worry about that," Elaine said. Then turning to her husband, she said, "I'll stay if you wish, Honey. You can go home." *Was that a sigh of relief I heard? He was off the hook.* With that matter sorted out, I caught up with Emily's immediate care, and then started on Lindsey.

* * *

Behind Lindsay's simple exterior, there was a real little kid who had gotten short-changed in life, and was now was unable to do anything for herself. It was unlikely that she recognized many of the staff, but she could identify her family and other familiar faces, and was happy when they visited her. She was relaxed. Daytime and nighttime were all the same to her when she was in the PedsICU. Because of increased secretions, she endured repeated suctioning though her little trach which caused her to cough and gag. G-tube feedings, medications, and the occasional sore butt and infections were her lot. This was her life. The days passed by monotonously. Her family knew that eventually she would be placed in a home for fragile kids –but not yet. They were not ready for her to leave them, forcing them to cope with the emptiness and guilt that was sure to follow.

CHANGING PLACES

I fed and medicated Lindsey through the G-tube and then bathed her. I didn't want a redo of last night's shenanigans with Kevin. Then, rolling her onto the sling, I winched her up and weighed her. While Lindsey swung in the air, I changed the linen and then slowly let her back down onto the clean bed, re-positioned her and suctioned her trach one more time. That done, I tidied her room and slid the door almost closed, satisfied that I had completed a significant part of my work for Lindsey for the night. *What must a lifetime of caring for Lindsey be like? Four nights in a row is enough for me.* And I turned my attention to Emily.

* * *

"M-o-m," I heard as I approached Emily's room. "M-o-m."

Emily's voice sounded more like that of a sickly 5-year-old kid than a pre-teen. Whiny. Insistent. Irritating. No sooner than the word had been uttered once, or twice –or maybe three times, than Emily's mom sprang from the recliner to her side saying, "What it is my Sweet?" or "I'm here, Emily." It wasn't yet 11 PM! *If*

Emily keeps the whining up, Elaine won't be jumping up with such alacrity in two hours —then whose turn will it be I wonder?

By midnight Emily's many whiny demands had become more than a little tiresome to me. "Mommy, I want a cool washcloth on my forehead." *Well – how about a please Emily?* "Mom, my nose is itching. Scratch it." *Scratch it yourself, Emily. The surgery was on your back, not your fingers.* "M-o-m, change the TV channel." *How about you doing that Emily? That's what's a remote is for.* "Mom –I want more ice chips…I'm thirsty…Give me a drink."

Elaine plied Emily with soothing responses, washcloths, ice chips and cartons of juice, tending to Emily's every request. "How do you feel Emily, my Sweet?" "Do you have any pain, Emily?" "Here's another cran-grape juice, Emily. You love cran-grape." "Have you given yourself some pain medication recently Emily?"

To which Emily would reply, "N-o-oo, Mom. Where's my clicker?"

I popped in and out of the room, checking on Emily's status, hanging medications and making sure that everything was going smoothly. Occasionally I reminded Emily to push the PCA button if she was experiencing pain. "You'll feel a whole lot better in the morning, after a good night's rest," I assured Emily. I stood at the bedside chatting to Elaine as Emily pushed the button again, and drifted back to sleep.

"Elaine, don't worry about Emily's medication," I reminded her. "She can't over-dose herself, and if the reverse happens, and it doesn't give her enough pain-relief, I can up the dose by re-programming it —within the prescribed parameters, of course." Elaine was relieved. "And if the worse comes to the worse, and Emily maxes-out on the dose, the surgeon will re-evaluate her need for better pain relief in the morning – and may even increase the dose further. He could even change the medication, if needs be."

"That's good to know. Emily has a low pain threshold," Elaine reminded me. *Of course she has.*

"It's just that you need some sleep Elaine, and I don't want you to worry. I really can take care of Emily," *even though I quite enjoy you doing so.* And I went back to the station, leaving Elaine and Emily just visible in the beams of the dim, night light and from the reflections of the overhead monitors.

By 2 AM, having had to get out of the recliner several times an hour, it was beginning to takes a toll on Elaine. *Perhaps Emily is like this at home.* I got on with my charting, glad that Elaine was sitting right beside Emily. Elaine was holding up well –better than I would be if Emily was my kid. *But then if Emily was my kid, she would not be asking for all the stuff in the first place! Duh!*

* * *

Mandy was an excellent nurse, popular with the patients, their families, and the other nurses. She had a reputation for being a bit goofy at times, but her kindness and thoughtfulness more than made up for that. I was sure every kid would want Mandy to be their nurse, if they could choose.

Mandy had looked after Kevin before and knew what kind of night to expect. She got stuck into her work, and by 11 PM, she too had gotten one of her patients settled. That left John.

I continued charting. Catch-up-charting was usual after an admission. I noticed Mandy walk into John's room. There had been a steady stream of visitors in and out of his room. *He sure hasn't been short on visitors. Good.*

They had been well-dressed, young adults, except for one or two older people. *Grandparents?* A couple of times I glanced through the crack in the curtains and saw John sitting quietly on the side of his bed. He looked as though he was about 4-years-old and had an unruly mop of thick, dark auburn curls. By 11 PM, John's last visitor had left, and Mandy proceeded to chart too.

"Is anyone staying the night with your kid?" I asked Mandy, looking in John's direction.

"I don't think so," she replied. "I think they've all gone for the night. His dad is staying in a motel nearby, with John's brother and sister."

While I did not need to know *all* about John, I needed to know a little about him, for when Mandy took her break, or was away from the station, it was vital that I could make safe decisions for her patients. Kevin wasn't a problem –but John was new. "So, what's up with your kid in there?" I asked innocuously. "He looks like a cute little boy." I paused. "What happened? There sure have been a lot of visitors. Is he doing okay?"

"It's sad," Mandy said. *Not another horrible disaster.* The pit of my stomach began to churn.

"John was in an accident today, a car accident...and his mom was killed." *That is terrible news.* We heard that somebody died in an MVA much too often in the PICU: adults dying, brothers, sisters or friends dying, and then the inevitable —our kids dying, and not making it to the PICU. Sometimes the child made it onto the unit, and someone very important to them, didn't. Very tough. Despite advice from Social Workers, Chaplains and nursing staff concerning the importance of honesty with kids, some families still played little games with their kids when a family member had died. We were left to follow, doing our best to be honest.

"If Julie asks how Sarah is, tell her she is at home getting better." *Nah... I don't think so.* You can couch the truth a little, and shield them from the gory, naked truth surely —but blatant lies?

"Tell him that Poppa will be in to see him in a few days. Poppa's got an owie!" *Oh please. They're going to find out, and won't like it that you lied to him.* Telling tall stories about where parents were, or how they were, made the nurse's job more stressful, especially if the child was alert, old enough, and well enough to ask real questions that needed real answers.

CHANGING PLACES

Assuaging my conscience with the rationale that I was asking Mandy questions on a need-to-know basis, I started a barrage of questions despite it not being exactly my business. But, I didn't want to be the one to confuse John inadvertently. He wasn't my patient, and I would have to play along with the family, whatever the case may be.

"Who was driving the car?...Was his dad in the car?...What about the rest of John's family?...Was anyone else killed?" And the final question, "Does John know his mom died?"

"John's mom was the only one to die in the accident," Mandy said. "Someone jumped a red light and ...bam... they were T-boned. John's grandpa is on another unit, and he's pretty ill. He'd been driving, and thankfully everyone was wearing their seatbelts."

"It could have been a lot worse if they hadn't," I said.

"And yes, John's dad told him that his mom is dead. I don't know who broke the news to his dad. Probably the CHP." *How sad* –and then the cogs started turning in my brain. *Well, for crying out loud, why isn't anyone staying with*

John tonight? Why isn't anyone holding his little hand...stroking his head...hugging and kissing him...and telling him everything will be okay? Where is his family now?

And the night wore on.

***

Six hours after returning from PSIF surgery, patients are log-rolled for the first time. That is a significant activity for the new post-op patient, but an important, necessary step in their recovery. The continued two-hourly turning routine of rolling the patient from one side to the other while keeping their spine in perfect alignment, was part of post-op care, and could not be avoided. But it was not a job for one nurse to tackle on her own, especially the first time.

"I need turners in Room 15," I called over the intercom. I had already instructed Elaine as to how to help in this maneuver, but reinforcements were needed.

Ellen, the Charge Nurse, was quick to come and Mandy put down what she was doing, to help with the big turn. Emily was awake and noticed the lights go up.

"Don't hurt me —Mommy, don't let them hurt me," she cried.

Tell the truth, Tabitha.

"Emily…we have to turn you now —and it's going to hurt. Did you give yourself some medication a few minutes ago?"

"Y-e-s," she wailed. "But will it hurt?"

She was almost crying now.

"Yes, Emily, it will hurt, but we have to do it. I have two nurses to help me —and your mom. She's going to help too. You must hang tough. You'll get through it. The first turn is the worst. You can do it."

Then I went into over-drive.

"Ellen and Mandy, will you go to the right of the bed?" I directed. "I'll pull Emily towards me and take care of her on this side, and you can be the stuffers. There are four pillows over there on the chair. And Mom?" I said, turning to Elaine who was standing by the recliner, "All you need to do is hold Emily's hand —next time we will make you work harder!" I continued with the plan. "Ellen, you do the pillows between her legs, and Mandy, the back pillows. Is that okay?" I had strategically placed three extra pillows ready for use.

"Okay guys," I continued as though marshaling a regiment, and not just two nurses and a nervous mother, "On the count of three.... One. Two. Three," and I heaved Emily firmly and smoothly up onto her left side. She screamed.

"Oh, I forgot Ellen, check her dressing please." Ellen checked the long dressing that extended from Emily's neck to her buttocks.

"No leakage. Looks great. Drains aren't kinked" Ellen reported, and she and Mandy each stuffed a pillow along Emily's back. Emily let out a cry with each push of the pillows and I hung onto the bath blanket, keeping her on her side. "Let her down now, Tabitha," Ellen said.

I carefully let go of the sheet allowing Emily to lean back onto the pillows while, at the same time, Mandy went to the foot of the bed and lifted Emily's right leg just enough for me to slide a pillow between her legs.

We all stood up. "There," I cooed, "how's that Emily? ... It wasn't too bad was it?" Emily did not reply. "You sure did well," I added.

It was the truth, for it could have been much worse. Mandy lavishly praised Emily for being a good kid, and everyone exited her room leaving Emily with her mom, who went back to watching television. Mission accomplished, time to chart. "Remember to click the clicker," I said as I left the room.

I positioned myself so that I could see the monitors for both Emily and Lindsey, and checked my notes for what still had to be done. Time passed, and Emily called out for her mom who was dozing in the recliner. I changed, turned, suctioned and fed Lindsey, and Mandy cared for Kevin. John drifted off to sleep after being given an analgesic for his injuries.

* * *

Time passed slowly. Mandy still needed to bathe and weigh John. That was the night shift's job for young kids, but she let him sleep. Waking him up, only for him to remember the awful reality that his mom was dead and never coming back, was something Mandy would not do for the sake of a few checkmarks.

By 2.30 AM John was awake, sitting up in bed, and crying. Mandy slipped into his room and sat down at the side of his bed, giving him more medicine to ease the pain. Almost 100 tiny stitches kept his ear in place, and his right hand also had many stitches in it. His bruised face and hand were very swollen, and no-doubt fear, sadness, and inner confusion tormented him.

I watched Mandy move and sit beside John, who sat cross-legged in his bed. Mandy had her arm around him. He was crying softly. As I kept watch at the station, Mandy then helped John select a favorite movie, and they began to watch it together in the quiet of the night hours. They looked so cute and relaxed, that for a short while I forgot the harsh reality of what was hidden from sight.

* * *

By 3 AM Emily had worn her mom to a frazzle. Elaine had finally fallen asleep in the chair. Wet washcloths dangled from Emily's bed rails and empty juice cartons littered her bedside table. The monitors clicked —relentlessly, lulling them both into a restful sleep. The PCA pump showed minimal usage.

John's medicine did not work the magic it had the first time around. He didn't fall asleep, so Mandy decided to bathe him, weigh him, and then see if that would do the trick and send him into la-la-land again. I went in to help Mandy with the scales and bed linen change. That job completed, Mandy stayed with John until he settled down and began to drift off to sleep. "I'll be right outside your door, John," Mandy told him as she opened the curtains a little, so that John could see the Nurses Station in the dim light. Soothing antibiotic ointment on the torn, reddened skin and road-rash, coupled with more analgesic medication, started to take effect, and he relaxed once more, falling to sleep again.

"Did you know, Tabitha, that he hasn't said one word to me the whole shift?" Mandy asked me. "Poor little mite. He must be numb with shock. He's so cute." She paused. "I wish we could make it right for him." *I wish that too, with all my heart.*

"By the way, Mandy, how come no one stayed with John tonight?" I asked. "It must be awful for him. He needs someone he knows with him. You are a great nurse Mandy —and I'm sure John feels safe with you, but you aren't family. He doesn't really *know* you. Don't they realize how traumatizing this could be for him? He's in pain, in hospital and alone. Wouldn't you be scared?"

Mandy and I discussed the situation remembering other sad times, but there was no real solution. Tonight it was John. Another night, it would be another kid. We could only imagine what it must be like to have a mother die when she was within touching distance. The screeching brakes. The force of the impact. The sirens. A cacophony of sounds. Being tightly strapped to a backboard. Scary IVs. Horrific pain. Confusion. And now ticking quietness in a strange place.

"I wonder if he thinks he's going to die."

***

I thought that Emily had probably nominated me already for the "The Most-Mean Nurse Award." Elaine was clapped-out in the recliner, next to Emily. She was fast asleep. *The next time Emily calls I am going to put things into perspective for her. It just might make things a little better. At least it won't make matters worse,* and I continued charting.

CHANGING PLACES

The station was silent as the monitors clicked monotonously in the background. It was 4 AM when, from the dark recesses of Room 15, came the familiar whining tones, "M—o—m?" Elaine didn't stir.

I was up in a flash. The chair skidded out from beneath me and across the station as I dashed soundlessly, into Emily's room.

"Emily...what do you want?" I asked as gently as I could.

"I want a drink," she whined, but before Emily could call her mom to give her the drink, I launched myself into The Talk, pleading her mother's case. "Emily...your mom is right here beside you. She is not going to leave you, but you must realize she is worn out. She does not have the energy to stay awake all night. You must let her rest. I know you would prefer your mom do everything for you, but for the time being, I'll do what you need to have done. Let your mom sleep for a few hours. She needs some rest. Yesterday was a long, stressful day for her, and you're big enough to understand how exhausted she must be. Just let her rest."

PEDIATRIC ICU 101

Giving a straight talk to a kid was not most PICU nurses' favorite job. But how else would our patients learn? I always wanted to alert the whiniest, most recalcitrant kids, to a different, more thoughtful way of thinking. I knew that I had been palmed off with a few of those difficult kids over the years, as well as some of the more troublesome families, because word had gotten around that if anyone could sort them out, Tabitha could. It was true that I often could —but not always. The cure came about through the mix of my formal Queen's English accent, and my down-to-earth, no-nonsense attitude. Or perhaps, I just put the fear of God into the kids, which made them reformed characters for the duration of their stay on the unit —or at least to the end of my shift.

After I had given Emily another cool washcloth and a drink, I turned to leave. Elaine slept peacefully in the recliner by Emily's bed. It was against the rules for parents to sleep at the bedside, but then rules had to be bent sometimes. Even I agreed with that.

Suddenly my mind went into overdrive, and I re-opened the door I was closing. "Emily, I can't tell you much, but I want you to know that you are *very* fortunate to have your mom right here, beside you, and a dad who loves you. Take it from me —you really are a very fortunate young lady. Thanks for giving your mom a break. She deserves that."

* * *

It was ironic that two kids could be geographically so close to one another, and yet have lives that were so dissimilar. *What would their lives look like in the future?* John would give up the world to change places with Emily if he could get his mom back for just one more hour. If only we could put John's clock back a day and have a re-do with a different ending, and put Emily's clock forward three-days, to a time when she would be up and walking, moderately pain-free. But, If Onlys are just that –If Onlys, and changing places wasn't an option.

PEDIATRIC ICU 101

CHAPTER 8

Speak Up, I'm Listening

IN THE '80s the PICU staff were required to attend a four-hour workshop on communication, at which I learned how to answer the telephone. I have the certificate to prove it.

"What you say is important," the speaker's syrupy voice drizzled over me. "You are a front-line employee. You are talking to the patient's family." She was in a different league from me. I had been taught to call a spade a shovel, and no amount of syrup could make my conversations into a perfect tête-à-tête which the perfectly-put-together instructor expected of me.

"You may be the first contact a person has with your place of work. Smile, as you answer the phone." *Yeah, right. Smile when I am changing a diaper with one hand, and holding the phone precariously under my chin as I listen to a concerned, or angry family member, at the other end of the line. Smile? I don't think so.*

Talking on the phone was not a priority in my childhood. We had a phone, but no one called my mother, and I certainly had no one to "ring." I saw my friends at school, and when school was over, I went home and would see my friends the next day, or the next week. What was there to say on the phone that I couldn't tell them then? And if I wanted to play with my friend next door, then I would go next door, knock on the door, and ask if I could play. Why pay for a phone call when I had perfectly good legs to use, and nothing to do with my time except homework, play the piano, take the dogs for a walk, ride my bicycle, or listen to the radio? It didn't make sense to me then, and it still wasn't of importance to me. They were wasting their money paying for me to go to the workshop, even though I probably was in desperate need of help! I just did not pick up on the importance of a good phone-voice.

Callers' lives are now more chaotic and stressful than ever, and health-dollars are in short supply, so employers aren't giving their work-force even a two-hour refresher course on communication skills for us to snooze, or chuckle, our way through. No more communication PowerPoints and role-plays for us. There is no money for such a luxury. However, being older and wiser, I know that communicating with our kids and their families can be extremely taxing, and wondered if I would have scored better in the communication department had I paid more attention at the workshop.

***

However, miscommunication can sometimes alleviate the seriousness of a shift.

Picture it. A parent walks up to the PedsICU door and peers through a long, narrow window in one of the doors. Sitting at a desk, about 20-feet down the hallway, partially hidden by a counter, she can see a harried lady on the phone. This lady is the Unit Secretary, who is usually busy, and usually female. Behind her, nurses move back and forth, steering IV poles, talking to colleagues on the phones, checking medications, disappearing from sight –only to dash across the scene in the opposite direction a few moments later. That is Station One, almost always busy.

The parent looks to her left and notices a doorbell, and an intercom system. Pressing the button twice, she sees Alvina, the unit secretary look up, and make eye contact with her. "Yes?" Alvina says "What can I do for you?" she asks in a pleasant voice, despite her obvious busyness.

"I want to see my baby," the woman replies.

Alvina has heard this one before, but knowing she is on the frontline, she smiles again and says gently, "And what is your baby's name?"

The woman replies "Jose."

"Jose?" Alvina repeats.

"Si," says the visitor.

The whiteboard to the left of the secretary lists only patients' last names, so Alvina speaks into the microphone head while working on a bunch of orders scribbled in the open chart on her desk. Typed orders are a rarity at this time, although, typed Order Sets are relatively common for specific diagnoses and procedures.

"Jose who?"

The visitor has now mastered the intercom button, and says, "Jose Hernandez."

Competent secretaries know that tracking down a kid, or his nurse, can be a long process. In this case, there are two Hernandezes, with "Name Alert" stickers beside them. Alvina presses the intercom button once more.

"How old is Jose?" she asks, and waits. The caller doesn't understand the question. "I will try to find out where he is. Are you wearing your armband?" Alvina asks, but the woman doesn't respond. All parents are required to wear armbands linking them to their child —a safety measure to protect their child. Alvina checks a more comprehensive list of names taped to her desk, and finds Jose Hernandez is in Room 12. She calls into Jose's room over the intercom.

"Hello? Debra? Are you there?" Silence. Apparently she isn't, so Alvina re-dials, this time into the Nurses Station. *Ding-dong.* "Debra —is Debra there?"

Debra doesn't reply, but another nurse in Station Three says, "She's not here —Debra's in Room 11".

All the while charts pile up on Alvina's desk with complex, new orders to enter, pharmacy orders to fax, diagnostic tests to schedule and more. "Thanks," Alvina says, and is gone. Tracking nurses can take a while with 25-rooms on five stations.

The anguished visitor fidgets by the door, hoping for the best, but fearing the worst. Is Jose dead? Is the secretary stalling for time? What is happening?

Ding-dong. "Debra?" There is a pause. "Debra?"

This time another voice answers. Sabrina is the patient in Room 11, and her mom knows how the system works after 10-long-days at the hospital with her daughter. "Debra's gone out," she says. "I think she's at the Station."

Alvina decides to change tactics and telephone the Station. Four-one-nine-seven-six. *Ring-ring.*

SPEAK UP, I'M LISTENING

"Station Three. This is Debra,"

"At last Debra. Jose's mom is at the door. Can she come in?"

Debra checks the screen and looks into Jose's room. "Alvina... it can't be his mom —his mom's already here – and someone else –maybe a grandmother. Ask her who she really is?"

And so it goes on, until Jose's grandmother leaves the room, doing a switcheroo with the supposed mom at the door –who is really Jose's aunt.

What a kerfuffle for one visitor! No wonder unit secretaries weren't begging to work in PedsICU, however, had Alvina gone to the four-hour workshop on communication style, tracking nurses and interacting with visitors would not have been such a protracted nightmare for the front-liners, the unit secretaries, especially when PedsICU became a 24/7 lock-down unit.

* * *

"One day a visitor will be so upset at me for making them wait, that I'll be looking down the barrel of a loaded handgun on the other side of the door, and have no time to punch the panic button," Connie, a night-shift secretary said. A panic button was on every station, and there was one at the front desk. "It's okay for you nurses down at the other end of the unit, safe in your stations, but what about me? I'm on the frontline." She was right. She was on the proverbial frontline, and who could know what an irate parent would do next.

One matter locked-doors partially resolved was that they concealed the flow of expletives volleying out of angry visitors' mouths when we asked them to wait a little longer, or perhaps, the annoyance of the locked-doors increased the problem –but, in either case we could hardly hear the expletives.

"I'm sorry, but the nurse is still busy, sir ... you will have to wait a little longer...I will get back to you." *Click*.

One day, this request was one time too many for a tall, white, shaven-headed, tattooed, visitor who glared at the secretary through the glass. He let rip a succession of curse words about the secretary and the nurses, that would shock the hardiest sailor. However, unknown to him and his family, not only were they visible from the desk through CCTV, but microphones picked up what was said for a short while after visitors heard the click of the phone. The man was in mid-flow of snide remarks and crude, rude comments, when a strong voice boomed out over the intercom above him saying, "If you use that language again, I will call security." The man stopped in mid-sentence and looked up in astonished guilt. It was as though he had heard the voice of God. Sitting by Connie, the Charge Nurse continued watching him.

"I just couldn't resist it," Connie said, "and thankfully he didn't have a loaded shotgun –this time."

* * *

An efficient communication system is essential in any ICU, and our unit-wide intercom allowed calls to go into one station, two or three stations, or between multiple floors at one time, depending on the operator's skill, and need. As soon as the familiar *ding-dong* rang out alerting staff to an up-coming message, voices quietened. Frequently an "all-call" request for equipment, a physician, or the Charge Nurse were made. It was a blessing, because the unit was vast, and no one had the desire or time to traipse around the floor unnecessarily.

Ding-dong, "Donnie, please dial zero-zero, Donnie" at which time Donnie dutifully pressed zero-zero, and connected with the caller. Other common messages were, *ding-dong,* "Dr. So-and-So, please come to the front desk for a transport call," or, *ding-dong,* "Anna, the transport has arrived," or occasionally, the more exciting message, *ding-dong* "the pot-luck is ready!"

Calling a Resident over the intercom at the beginning of his first rotation adds sparkle to a dreary shift, because it is likely that the new physician does not know how to answer an intercom call. Selectively using the intercom, can be a particularly poignant way of getting a physician who has already demonstrated a perceived superior, close-proximity to God, down to earth with a thud! After calling Dr. New-doctor over the intercom and hearing no reply, the nurse will make a more urgent call that get everyone's attention. *Ding-dong,* "Dr. New-doctor, *please* call back. Dr. New-doctor."

Nurses near him get a kick out of watching Dr. New-Doctor's flummoxed behavior, as he tries to answer the intercom before another embarrassing request for his help is broadcast unit-wide. Having to ask a lowly nurse how to answer the intercom, is a humbling experience. *Welcome, Dr. New-Doctor to the Team.*

SPEAK UP, I'M LISTENING

Intentionally misusing the intercom system is unprofessional, and should not be done as it is impossible to know who is on the floor, and if serious discussions are going on between our physicians and some parents, but inevitably, stumbled communications occur when a new, or nervous nurse, is forced to use the intercom. Embarrassed by again giving a garbled message for all to hear, she swears she will never use the system again, until she has to. It is inevitable that every nurse will say something stupid over the intercom at some time, and, if she dares to think she would never be so foolish, beware, pride goes before a fall, or so King Solomon says.

* * *

Justin, an experienced, well-liked PICU nurse, had a very critical kid and needed another med-fusion pump, a small device that delivers IV medications accurately to patients in minute quantities. It was a quiet night when he spoke into the inter-com.

Ding-dong. "Does anyone have a med-fusion pump? If you do, dial zero-zero". *Duh...what nurse didn't have a med-fusion pump?* Every kid had one or two med-fusion pumps at their bedside, and very critical kids may have as many as five med-fusion pumps ticking beside their bed at one time. Unused pumps left at Nurses Stations were quickly spirited away by eagle-eyed staff, and concealed, "just in case." After Justin had unintentionally omitted the word "extra", a kindly nurse ignored his error, and brought him a pump from her hidden stash. However, the rest of the night was set for jokes on Justin about med-fusion pump availability as they passed his room.

"Justin, 24 of the patients on the floor have med-fusion pumps. Why hasn't your kid got one?"

"Justin, who is Anyone?"

"Justin, there are two med-fusion pumps in the shower, in the staff restroom. I hid them there, just in case."

Justin took the ribbing with style, smiling and laughing his way through the shift, but the following night, nurses thought twice before calling for a med-fusion pump, and carefully watched Justin as he was likely to give as good as he got!

***

SPEAK UP, I'M LISTENING

Visitation rules were posted in both English and Spanish beside the intercom microphone outside the PedsICU in full view of potential rule-breakers. There had to be no excuses for visitors not to know what was expected of them. Kids under 14 were kids, not adults, and could not visit freely. This rule helped prevent cross-infection between our kids, and visiting kids who had common childhood illnesses. We sure did not want our kids catching another infection to add to their already ill disposition, nor did we want to give a virulent infection to a young visitor. Smart rule. Nevertheless, some families balked at it.

Visitors snuck through the doors by closely following others who had received permission to come in, or they came in behind a member of staff. However, unit secretaries had an uncanny way of seeing the invisible, and as the uninvited visitor was about to swish past the front desk, they would hear, "Hello...can you wait here, please? Are you with this family? Just wait please." Then, depending on the outcome of the "interrogation", the sneaker-in may be refused entry, and sent back down the long hall to the swing-doors in humiliation, to wait their turn. Foiled, or perhaps allowed in.

Or maybe a kid sneaks in. "Hi there, Son. Visiting your sister?" the secretary will ask the kid who is trailing in behind his mom. *The visiting child cannot possibly be 14 years old.*

"Yes," the kid says as his mother continues down the hall, anxious to get to her child's room.

"What year were you born, Son?" the secretary asks and, before the kid can work out what year he should answer had he been 14 years old, the wrong answer is out.

"I'm sorry, young man. You need to be 14 to visit without seeing a Child Life Specialist. Your mom must make an appointment for you to see Child Life Specialist before you can come in. You will have to turn around, and wait outside."

That is front-line work!

* * *

Interviewing siblings is only part of the Child Life Specialists work-a-day. At scheduled appointments, often in a special play room, CLSs use age-appropriate communication and play for visiting siblings before they go into their brother's or sister's room. The daunting environment of an ICU room can be overwhelming for many kids, especially if their sibling is likely to die. The visitors' immunization records are reviewed, and any contact with infectious diseases should be disclosed, as should recent illnesses. This is for everyone's health and safety. Then, when the visiting child first sees their very ill sibling, they have with them a kindly, knowledgeable host, who will answer all their questions. This is helpful to the visiting child, the family, the patient and of course, the nursing staff.

Our patients love Child Life Specialists because they bring age-appropriate activities to children's bedsides, and will even play with them when they are lonely or bored. The CLS also have a vast library of DVDs and video games, X-boxes and more, to lend to our kids. Our kids get personal visits from the CLS, whereas kids on the Basic Pediatric Floors enjoy scheduled sessions in the Play Rooms, where no medical interventions are allowed. That's a rule, and keeps the play rooms happy, safe places for the little patients.

***

Communication is important, whether you are a Unit Secretary on the front frontline, a nurse talking to her patient's parents face-to-face or over the phone, or calling a code over the intercom. Clear, kind communication makes life sweeter for everyone.

Families entering PedsICU don't notice minor gaffes over the intercom usually, and if they do, they overlook them because they know the nurses are diligent professionals who work with a team of healthcare providers whose collective goal is to get their child well again. This is what is most important to everyone, even when an amusing turn happens on PedsICU.

It is here, in the PICU, that medical science, emotional pain, stress and miracles go hand in hand, and where friendships run long and deep.

Glossary of Terms

acuities: calculations that determine the need for next shift's staff according to State regulations, based on the degree of illness of patients and the skill-level of nursing staff

ALOC: Altered Level Of Consciousness

AML: Acute Myelogenous Leukemia

analgesic: pain killer, pain medication

apneic spells: no breathing over a short period of time repeated occasionally

appy: abbreviation for *appendectomy*, excision of the appendix

PEDIATRIC ICU 101

Attending: Abbreviation for Attending Physician; a PICU Attending is also known as a Pediatric Intensivist

bradycardic spells: short periods of time when an infant's heart rate is critically slow

CMS: Circulation, Movement, Sensation

COPD: Chronic Obstructive Pulmonary Disease; serious lung conditions usually in found in adults

Dandy-Walker: Dandy-Walker Syndrome, DWS. Congenital brain malformation syndrome.

DNR: do not resuscitate; AKA "No Code"

ER: Emergency Room

extubated: removal of an endotracheal tube

febrile: feverish; a body temperature exceeding the normal of 37° C / 98.4°F

Float: (noun) a Float (nurse) works on a floor that is not her usual workplace; Floats may be hired to work a variety of floors regularly; **to float** (verb) to work for a shift, or short time in, a place other than a nurse's home-base unit. Nurse receives a differential usually

GLOSSARY OF TERMS

goober: slang for large, thick dollops of secretion, usually from the lungs

graduate: a triangular, measuring container

G-tube: gastrostomy tube; tube to deliver medications and feedings directly into the stomach through a surgically created opening in the abdominal wall

hemoc: abbreviation for "Hematology and Oncology", Hemoc Unit

herniate: bulging, prolapse of tissue; will cause death when brain tissue swells within a formed structure, the cranium, and therefore pushes downwards into the spinal column

HIPAA: Health Insurance Portability and Accountability Law 1996; provides for health information privacy

intubate: to place a breathing tube into the lungs through the mouth, or nose, in order to mechanically support breathing

Is & Os: intake and output; calculations made each shift, or more frequently, which include all fluids going into a patient (IV, oral etc.) and all output (urinary, through drains etc.) to provide an accurate fluid balance report

log-roll: moving a patient from one side to another without destabilizing the spine

looky-loos: people who stare at motor vehicle accidents causing delays or pile-ups; applied to inappropriate gawking at other patients

MVA: motor vehicle accident

NAT: Non-Accidental Trauma. Child is possibly admitted due to abuse

NICU: Neonatal Intensive Care Unit

No Code: resuscitation status where a parent, or the next of kin, have authorized no treatment should be provided should an emergency occur; the same as DNR

NPO: nothing by mouth.

Odd: a nurse's work list that is a single patient; a second patient may be added to that list during the shift if the first patient's condition improves

one-to-one: one nurse caring for one, high acuity patient, over a shift

OR: operating room

GLOSSARY OF TERMS

OSHA: Occupational Safety and Health Administration; an agency of the US government responsible for safety at work and a healthful work environment

PB: personal best —as in sports

PCA: Patient Controlled Analgesia; a computerized, intravenous analgesic delivering device set to provide prescribed doses of analgesia, usually post operatively, by patients, to themselves

peds: (pronounced "peeds") abbreviation for "pediatric"

Prader-Willi: Prader Willi Syndrome; genetic disorder which causes a child to be constantly hungry

residuals: process of aspirating liquids in the stomach via an artificial means, measuring it, and possibly refeeding it

RSV: Respiratory Syncytial Virus; a common respiratory infection usually affecting infants up to 2-years that may cause pneumonia, bronchiolitis or death (in severe cases) if not treated

RT: Respiratory Therapist

SCDs: Spontaneous Compression Devices; devices placed around a patient's leg calves to maintain venous blood flow post-operatively, or when a patient is incapacitated for a long period of time

septic: condition of sepsis

Step-down: abbreviation for Step-Down Intensive Care Unit which provides less specialized care than an Intensive Care Unit but more intense care than does a Basic Unit

Supe: (pronounced "soup"), Supervisor

switcheroo: jargon to describe switching visitor(s) already at a bedside out, for another visitor waiting to come in

TPN: Total Parenteral Nutrition; a highly nutritious form of intravenous fluid. usually given through a central line

trach: abbreviation for "tracheostomy"; artificial opening into the windpipe, surgically effected

Yankauer: a strong, large bore suction catheter for thick, or excessive, oral secretions

About the Author

TABITHA B. C. ABEL lived a quiet life in the English countryside with her mother and sister Rebecca, who was 19-months her elder. Earlier, her father and mother lived the life of the rich (and not famous) in India for 20 years but when the marriage soured, Tabitha's mum returned to England where Tabitha was born. Her parents divorced when she was two, in the 1950s. Her mum was on her own with two young children and life wasn't easy. The three older children soon became adults and, receiving no financial support from anywhere, her mother was left to fend alone for the youngest children – despite her family's wealthy, aristocratic, heritage.

Tabitha became a nurse by default, and trained at King Edward VII Hospital in Windsor, Berkshire. Marrying a pastor in her early twenties, she became a State Certified Midwife at Halifax General Hospital in Yorkshire, and practiced as a midwife for the next nine years as they moved to different locations in the north of England. They had three children who are now adults, and still very important to her life.

Two significant milestones altered Tabitha's life forever. First, in the early 1970s, Rebecca, her sister, died in Queens, New York while she was with a friend on Christmas break. That incident introduced Tabitha to death at close hand, and dealing with loss. Rebecca had a full scholarship for graduate studies at Andrews University in Berrien Springs, Michigan. Later, in the early 1980s, and again in the early 1990s, Tabitha and her first husband moved between the UK and the US for study, and for her husband to work as a pastor and counsellor. Those were busy years and uprooting their young family three times to cross The Pond, to live in very different cultures, was another kind of trauma.

While in southern California, Tabitha worked at Loma Linda University Children's Hospital and in the

ABOUT THE AUTHOR

Medical Center, and studied at Loma Linda School of Public Health, eventually gaining a Master's degree in Health Promotion and a Doctoral degree in Public Health, Health Education. Later she earned a Master's degree in Nursing Education, from the University of Phoenix.

Tabitha felt privileged to work with an amazing team of nurses, physicians and medical professionals who tolerated her quirkiness in the various roles she filled in PedsICU from bedside nurse, to relief Charge Nurse, to potluck planner and editor of the monthly news-sheet, *PICK-U PostIt* –and general agitator (and encourager). Some of those people became her life-long friends and life moved on with her caring for other kids, in other locations, over a long career in nursing.

Despite her busy life as a mother –and less-than-perfect wife, student, nurse, and university and college adjunct faculty, Tabitha flourished under pressure and delighted in many friendships but, after a painful divorce, life went on, her children grew up and made their own life stories.

Divorce, as a Christian, is never pretty and brought a lot of regrets but now, married to her second husband,

Gary, she faces problems of another kind, as we all do. She still relies on God to get her through challenges today and now, retired from teaching and nursing, she continues to participate in short, and medium-term mission projects. She still remains a competitive runner and triathlete, and is a free-lance writer, musician, hiker and weekly blogger at Tabel Talk@TabithaBCAbel on Facebook.

Tabitha believes that one of the most incredible stories in the Bible is that of Jesus being invited to go to the home of a synagogue ruler because his 12-year-old daughter was ill. As they journeyed to her home, she died, and by the time they got to the house, the mourners were creating a racket and wailing loudly. This turned to jeers when Jesus said that the girl wasn't dead, but asleep. Ignoring the crowds, He, three of His disciples and the parents, went to the child's room where Jesus took her by the hand and said, "Little girl, arise." And she did. She came back to life (Mark 5:22-24, 35-43; Luke 8: 41, 42, 49-56)!

Tabitha wishes that the Great Physician would walk through every PedsICU and pediatric floor, and heal all

ABOUT THE AUTHOR

the kids. If only. But as His hands, she accepts the call to do her part, while waiting for a better time to come.

The KIDS IN CRISIS trilogy is long over-due for publication, especially KIDS IN CRISIS –Pediatric ICU 101. Tabitha firmly believes that the stories contained in each of the books will open reader's eyes to a world that they may never enter and help them to better understand what goes on behind those closed doors. The books are memoirs, written to provide readers with an educational, human-interest perspective on PICU nursing and are expected to fill a void in the present medical literature about caring for critically ill children.

Made in the USA
Lexington, KY
21 September 2019